MATRONS, MEDICS AND MALADIES

Matrons, Medics and Maladies

INSIDE EDINBURGH ROYAL
INFIRMARY IN THE 1840s

Bill Yule

DRAWINGS BY
JOHN JOHNSTONE

'I find the medicine worse than the malady.'
JOHN FLETCHER, 1579–1625
The Lovers' Progress

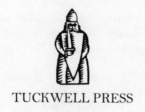

TUCKWELL PRESS

First published in Great Britain in 1999 by
Tuckwell Press, The Mill House, Phantassie,
East Linton, East Lothian EH40 3DG, Scotland

Copyright © Bill Yule 1999

ISBN 1 86232 091 8

British Library Cataloguing in Publication Data
A catalogue record for this book is available
on request from the British Library

Typeset by Antony Gray
Printed and bound by The Cromwell Press,
Trowbridge, Wiltshire

To my wife

Contents

Acknowledgements

Many people helped with this book. In particular I would like to thank Mike Barfoot, archivist of the Lothians Health Services Archive in Edinburgh University who allowed me to consult the records in his care. The help of the University's archivist, Arnott Wilson, is much appreciated as is that given by the staff of the Special Collections section of the University Library. Joan Auld, the archivist of Dundee University, set in motion the research that was eventually to lead to this book. To her enthusiasm I owe a great deal. Sadly she was killed in a climbing accident while the work was at an early stage. Patricia Whatley, Joan's successor, has been equally helpful, as have her staff and the librarians of Dundee University Medical School at Ninewells Hospital.

I have much pleasure in thanking my family. My daughter Katy spent much time finding bits of paper I had lost. My daughter Rosemary enjoyed commenting bluntly on what I had thought were apposite quotations. My wife Kirsty helped in many ways and provided Hebridean common sense when problems arose. I am grateful to them all.

The following are thanked for permission to use the material over which they have copyright.Full details of each source can be found in the bibliography.

Weidenfeld and Nicolson for permission to quote from Professor Geoffrey Best's *Mid-Victorian Britain*; Myrtle Simpson per John Johnson (Authors' Agent) Limited to use material from *Simpson the Obstetrician*; Churchill Livingstone for permission to quote from Lloyd and Coulter's *Medicine in the Navy, 1200-1900*, Volume 3; Churchill Livingstone for permission to quote from John Shepherd's *Simpson and Syme of Edinburgh*; Peters, Fraser and Dunlop, Writers' Agents, on behalf of the Estate, for permission to quote from Hilaire Belloc's 'Henry King' in *Cautionary Verses* published by Random

House UK Ltd; Longmans for permission to quote from A. T. Thomson's *Elements of Materia Medica and Therapeutics;* The *British Medical Journal,* the *Lancet* and the *Scottish* (formerly the Edinburgh) *Medical Journal,* Paul Harris for permission to quote from *Low Life in Victorian Edinburgh;* Professor Matthew Kaufmann for permission to quote from an article in the Edinburgh University Magazine *Edit.*

While every effort has been made to secure permission, it has in a few case proved impossible to trace an appropriate person or persons. Apologies are offered to anyone who thinks they should have been included and they are invited to contact the author or the publisher of this book.

Introduction

This book is not a ponderous, carefully balanced history of a great British hospital. It represents only one view of the Royal Infirmary of Edinburgh. The time is the 1840s.

The book has two aims. The first is to provide a sort of nineteenth century 'fly on the wall' documentary, using drawings instead of television, to follow the progress through the wards of those people who turned up unwell on the hospital's doorstep. The second is to make use of the 'social history' content of each patient's case notes. When this is put together with material from other contemporary sources a picture emerges of the lives of the staff and patients of the Infirmary, both in the hospital and outside in the lively streets of Edinburgh.

The main source material for this book remains just as it was written over one hundred and fifty years ago. It consists of the Royal Infirmary's original Ward Journals, long narrow volumes in which junior doctors kept detailed records of each patient's management and day-by-day progress. The Infirmary was run by a board of management whose minute books provide additional information about the people of the hospital. They also show the board at work, dealing with a wide range of problems, some serious, some quaint, and some amusing.

Why choose the 1840s? First because the original material just described is more complete at that time. All the large leather-bound volumes of the minutes, for example, have survived. With the clinical records they now form part of the Lothians Health Services Collection in Edinburgh University.

Second because it was an interesting decade in the city. There were really two Edinburghs. The New Town was increasingly prosperous. In 1841, for example, Charles Dickens was entertained in great style. The historian Anderson noted: 'A public dinner was given by the city council for Charles Dickens. Two hundred and fifty gentlemen were invited, added to in the evening by two hundred ladies who graced the event with their presence'. Dickens had a genuine sympathy for the poor and had already pointed out that 'the same world of emotion beats in their breasts as in the higher class'. Had he walked up the hill after dinner that night, he would have found a different world. The poverty-stricken people of the Old Town lived in as crowded and degrading conditions as were to be found in Britain. The extent to which this exposed them to epidemic disease, compared to their fellow citizens north of Princes Street, is discussed later.

The third reason for choosing the 1840s is because it was a lively time in the medical world. James Young Simpson and his friends and family first enjoyed the effects of chloroform in his house at 52 Queen Street. And Robert Syme, a brilliant surgeon, was then at the peak of his success and continuing to tease the board of management. All the gossip and activity of Edinburgh's medical 'establishment' was relished by the medical press of Edinburgh and London.

From its records it is clear that Edinburgh Royal Infirmary was living up to its charter's requirement that it 'care for the sick and hurt poor of Edinburgh'. Although it all happened a long time ago, this book does make use of the actual medical records of real people. A lingering respect for medical confidentiality has led to the decision to change patients' names.

Finally, a word of caution. Young hospital doctors used to have a reputation for high-spirited activities when off duty. Their behaviour was often dealt with leniently on the grounds that much that they and the nurses had to cope with during their day's work was unpleasant. One or two case histories in this book reflect this and the last chapter opens with a warning!

A Note on the Prescriptions

Throw physic to the dogs, I'll none of it!

SHAKESPEARE, *Macbeth*

Human physiology was not well understood in the 1840s which meant that there was little logical basis for pharmacology and thera-peutics. Many prescribed substances were ineffective and some, such as antimony, were dangerous. They were all very enthusiastically written up in a little book by Henry Beasley. The title page reads:

THE BOOK OF PRESCRIPTIONS:
Containing
2900 Prescriptions
collected from the practice of the most
eminent physicians and surgeons,
English and Foreign.
Comprising also,
A COMPENDIOUS HISTORY OF THE MATERIA MEDICA
OF ALL COUNTRIES,
ALPHABETICALLY ARRANGED
and
Lists of the Doses of all Officinal or Established Preparations.
BY
HENRY BEASLEY

This source is referred to frequently in this book. Little is known of Beasley apart from the fact that, between 1842 and 1895, he produced three major series. These were: *The Pocket Formulary, The Book of Prescriptions* and *The Druggist's General Receipt Book.* Each went into several editions. Otherwise Beasley is a shadowy figure. His name is not in the medical register and he was not a member of the Pharma-ceutical Society. His enthusiastic approach to his subject can be seen in his comments on his contributors and their favourite prescriptions. He can be alarming, for example when advising on the treatment of syphilis in children. He suggests spreading diluted mercurial ointment on a flannel roller, which is then to be wrapped round one leg. 'This', he adds, 'cures syphilis without any inconvenience, whereas very few children recover to whom mercury is given internally.'

In addition to Beasley's book the *British Pharmacopoeia* of 1867 has been a useful source in interpreting the Edinburgh prescriptions. This was the second edition of the BP, an amalgamation of the separate pharmacopoeias of England, Edinburgh and Dublin, put together by a small committee which included Christison of Edinburgh.

As the Infirmary's young doctors wrote up the case notes which form a large part of this book they used contemporary units such as drachms, minims, and scruples. Usually they wrote these as symbols. Here these symbols have been replaced by the full names of each unit. The unit of length known as a 'line' is referred to from time to time. This was one-twelfth of an inch.

MATRONS, MEDICS AND MALADIES

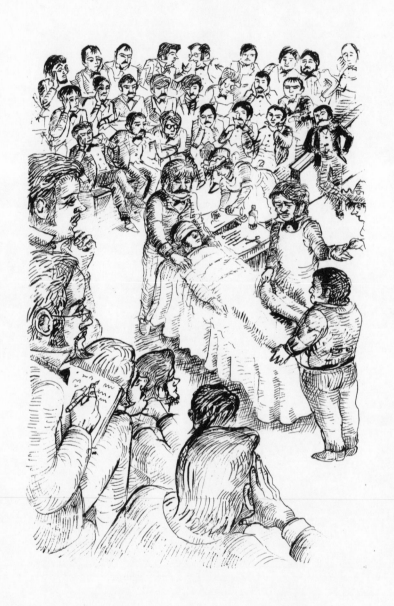

✣ 1 ✣

The Layout of the Infirmary
with a note on its history

Don't clap too hard – it's a very old building.

JOHN OSBORNE, *The Entertainer*

'The body of the House [i.e. the Infirmary] is 210 feet in length, from each end of which, and at right angles, a wing is extended 20 feet. There are three floors and an attic. On the third is a consultation room for physicians and surgeons and a waiting room for students. In the attic is a large theatre in which upwards of 200 students can at once see operations. Over the theatre is a cupola. The attic may also be used as a chapel.

'On the ground floor are twelve cells for mad people, two kitchens, the apothecary's shop and a servants' room. Adjacent to the shop is the apothecary's room, a dining room and the matron's parlour which communicates with her bedroom directly above. In her parlour is a chest for books of account. The physicians' clerks, the surgeons' clerks and the apothecary's assistant have their rooms on different floors and are so located that they may be ready to assist any sudden call from the patients.

'Two hundred and twenty-eight patients may be accommodated, each in a distinct bed, with a press at its head for containing medicines and a chart. Half of the beds are for men. Medical patients are on first and second floors, surgical on the third to give increased access to theatre. Patients after operation can then be transported conveniently and without agitation from the theatre to the adjoining beds on either side.

'The great stair running up the middle of the building, being spacious, admits of street chairs, in which people are brought to the hospital with fractures, dislocations or dangerous wounds, so that

3

people can be carried to the wards without difficulty. Further, people lodged in the high part of the hospital enjoy constant fresh air and are free from the noise of the lower parts, both of which are considered of importance to those who have undergone dangerous operations. On this, the third floor also, is a ward for lying-in women, sufficiently separate from the rest of the House and under the direction of a professor of midwifery [In the 1840s this was James Young Simpson]. Above this are extensive garrets in which many patients might be accommodated, but as heat or cold in them cannot be properly regulated, they are normally store rooms.

'On the other stairs and in a remote part of the House is a salivating ward for women containing twelve beds. This ward, being under the management of a prudent nurse, is never open but when she herself is present so that these patients cannot have any contact with the other wards. A further small ward of four beds is used for the same purpose but to accommodate women who, not from any fault of their own but from their husbands and sickly infant children, had applied to be cured in the hospital. The physicians finding it improper to throw these patients into the company of others whose conduct and manners are less correct, and considering them as no less objects of compassion as any other patients in the House, represented the case to the managers who gave orders for this ward. [A 'salivating' ward was one for the treatment of patients with syphilis. This is explained in the chapter on VD.]

'In the west wing are one cold and one hot bath with dressing rooms. A door leads to these baths from the Great Court. These baths are intended for the people of the city, no patient in the hospital having at any time any admittance to them. In the east wing there is a bath for the patients of the House, so constructed that it may be used either as hot or cold.' [There was, therefore, one bath for two hundred and twenty eight patients.]

'To these quaint paragraphs [*sic*] are added descriptions of the laundry and mortuary arrangements with which we do not need to concern ourselves.'

A NOTE ON THE HISTORY OF THE INfiRMARY

The above is a description of the first Royal Infirmary of Edinburgh, the fine Adam building in which all the events described in this book occurred. It was situated near the Old College of the University, between Drummond Street and Infirmary Street, with Edinburgh's city wall forming one boundary.

The Infirmary came into existence because of the Royal College of Physicians of Edinburgh. The college was founded in 1681, largely through the influence of Sir Robert Sibbald, who also wished to form a medical faculty in the University. From its earliest days its members interested themselves in the care of the poor. At the college's third meeting, on 10 February 1682, two physicians were appointed 'to serve the poor of the city and suburbs'. More appointments were made and the physicians found their efforts to provide care hindered by the want of suitable accommodation and appliances. So, in 1725, the College proposed the foundation of an infirmary. A subscription list was opened and the target of £2000 was easily reached. On 6 December 1729 a 'small hired house' with six beds was opened, on a temporary basis. It stood at the head of Robertson Close which linked the Cowgate and Infirmary Street. Its good work, and the strong support of people like George Drummond, the city's Provost, and Alexander Monro, the first of the Edinburgh professors of that name, led to the granting of a Royal Charter in 1736 for a proper hospital on the site. The first Edinburgh Royal Infirmary opened its doors in December 1741 for the care, as the Charter says, of 'the sick and hurt poor of Edinburgh'. As time passed it became clear that more beds were needed, so when, in 1828, the old High School of Edinburgh moved from its site adjoining the Infirmary to the Calton Hill, the empty school became the Infirmary's surgical hospital. A link was built between the two buildings. The Infirmary's junior doctors found this link useful for access to late-night activities but the board of management eventually did what boards always do. On 31 March 1845 they 'admonished Dr Cameron for irregularity of hours in passing from the medical to the surgical hospital' and added, 'instructions are to be given that the door between the two hospitals be locked at midnight'.

In 1879 the whole hospital closed, being replaced by a new Edinburgh Royal on the Meadows. As this is being written the third Royal Infirmary is nearing completion on the south side of the city.

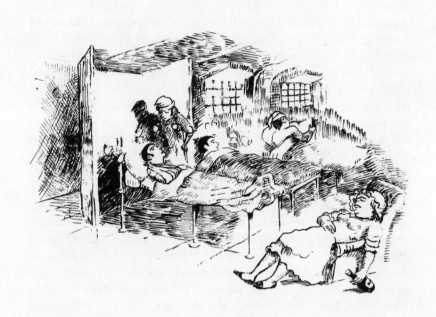

❦ 2 ❦

Nursing in the Royal Infirmary

The nurse sleeps sweetly, hir'd to watch the sick,
Whom, snoring, she disturbs.

COWPER

'Patients are, for several hours at a time, left entirely at the mercy of
the night nurses.' This surprising comment, taken from the Infirmary
board of management's minutes of 18 January 1841, sums up all that
was wrong with the 'old system' of nursing care in Edinburgh.

THE OLD SYSTEM

Things were certainly bad. On 18 January 1841, the managers
received a report from Mrs Wood, the matron, on the best way of
providing supervision of the Infirmary's nurses, especially at night.
She thought the day staff not too bad, although later they too were
seen as part of the notorious 'old system'. 'But', Mrs Wood wrote, 'it
is far otherwise with the night nurses. They are not only, when taken
as a whole, decidedly inferior in intelligence, and knowledge of their
duties, to the day nurses but at present are left to themselves the
greater part of the night without anyone to direct them or instruct
them. We are also unfortunately obliged to add that, although every
effort is made to induce respectable females to enter the service of
the Infirmary as nurses, scarcely a week passes over without the
dismissal of one or more of them for irregularities which cannot
be overlooked, the most frequent of which is drunkenness. The
managers could not at present confer a greater boon upon the
establishment than by placing the night nurses under some more
efficient superintendence.'

The board agreed and decided that the duties of those who were to
undertake the superintendence of the night nurses were to be two-
fold. First they were to see that the nurses were not asleep or absent

7

from the wards and that they were not burning too much gas or having too large fires in the wards. Secondly they were to see that the nurses 'do not drink the wine and spirits provided for the patients and, in very bad cases, that the wine and spirits prescribed are regularly given and in the quantities ordered'. The first requirement was to be achieved by irregular visits to the wards. The second needed sickbed experience in the supervisor. 'This will chiefly be needed in the fever wards, for, from the state of unconsciousness with which this disease when severe is generally accompanied, those patients are for several hours at a time left entirely at the mercy of the night nurses. When a patient is conscious, however, this acts a check upon negligence and culpability.'

The board offered the job on a trial basis to Mr Christie, the Apothecary's assistant, he being 'an active and trustworthy man who had medical training and knew doses of medicines. He is popular with the nurses and knows the hospital and its routine. A spare nurse is to be at his call to replace an unsatisfactory one. He will work in the apothecary's shop only in the morning and he will be paid an extra £30 per year.'

Christie tried the job but very quickly gave up. At the next board meeting on 7 February 1841, his resignation was accepted with regret. The matron said that it was not possible to get good night nurses for the fever wards 'especially as not a few had died in performing their duties, from being exposed to the influence of a contagious disease. They also have all the sheets and shirts of the ward to wash, and stairs and passages outwith the wards, leaving them inadequate time for patients.' The board responded by increasing the pay for nurses working in the fever wards and appointing another woman to wash the stairs and passages.

The attempt to provide supervision on an in-house basis having failed, it was decided to advertise for two night supervisors of nurses. This led to the appointment of Mrs McAndrew, matron of the Magdalen asylum, and a Mrs Smith. In October Mrs McAndrew found herself the subject of a complaint from a junior doctor, Richard McKenzie. He claimed 'that she, one of the supervisors of wards, had disturbed the patients in the night-time when finding fault with a nurse.' The board instructed her 'to be more circumspect' but failed to record that at least she was in the ward and checking-up on staff! But even these experienced women did not succeed. In December 1842 the board decided that the experiment of having superintendents of night nurses had been 'an utter failure.' Both were to be dismissed from Whitsun next unless suitable work was found for them elsewhere in the hospital. While it was agreed that some supervision of the nurses was needed, it had to be done 'much less expensively and much more efficiently.' There are no details of how this was achieved but at least the problems were now appreciated and the first steps along the thirty-year road to the 'new system' for Edinburgh Royal's nurses had been taken.

THE NEW SYSTEM

The school of nursing of the Edinburgh Royal Infirmary opened in 1872, the event marking the start of the 'new system'. Nursing now began to be seen as a profession instead of a poorly paid and unskilled task which attracted only the financially desperate and the altruistic. The change followed the Crimean War and the work of Florence Nightingale. Only then could it be claimed 'that a lady, whose inclination leads her to it, can be a probationer and a nurse in a great hospital without the loss of her self-respect, and without danger to her health. She can then lead a happy, useful and honourable life.'

This quotation is from an 1876 article in the *Edinburgh Medical Journal*. The writer heads his article 'Nursing in the Edinburgh Infirmary' and refers to himself as 'a former house surgeon in ERI.' 'Since the Crimean War,' he says, 'Florence Nightingale, by pen, influence and example, has done much to put the whole question of nurses and nursing on another footing. There are no Mrs Gamps now. No longer a coarse old beldame but an active, clever and a more conceited and lively young woman is the typical hospital nurse.'

He goes on: 'In what does this great change consist? First it was realised that nursing did not come to all women by intuition, that it was a difficult art requiring not only temper, firmness, obedience and that great faculty, capableness, but also that a certain amount of training rendered all those good qualities ten times more valuable. Secondly, such being the case, it gradually dawned upon the minds of hospital managers and doctors that such women need to be sought out. The old method of selecting hospital nurses seemed to be to accept at small wages all the domestic servants and widows who, from various reasons, did not get on in ordinary domestic service; the clever amongst them perhaps with bad temper or no character, the stupid either idle or shiftless. Some of them probably found their vocation and became valuable nurses, their value often eclipsed during a drinking bout, and being lessened by coarseness of speech. Others had their good qualities but with a fatal 'but'. For example, good tempered but lazy, kind and worthy but a hopeless slattern. Few could write a letter or answer a question intelligently.

'If the day nurses were largely inefficient, who shall tell the delinquencies of the poor old charwomen and scrubbers who were by courtesy called 'night nurses'? Worn out to begin with, underfed, underpaid, allowed five or six hours rest after a day of scrubbing before beginning a night of watching, what wonder was it that this watching was a farce and that she drowned her cares in whisky and laudanum and rested her weary back in any unoccupied bed in the ward? When the writer was a house surgeon, one of the duties of a really active doctor was to go round the ward during the mid-watch and rouse the night nurses! Hence for really urgent and severe surgical cases the dressers and house surgeons had to do the night nursing themselves.

'And over this unorganised crowd with no esprit de corps, the only superintendence was that of an already overworked housekeeper for whom the kitchen, the laundry and the storeroom were a heavy enough burden. The wonder is that things were not worse. On the old system, the day nurse was cook and housekeeper as well as nurse. The night nurse was drudge and scrubber, and only incidentally had to take on the difficult and trying work of nursing twenty sick and often dying men.

'The change to the new system came when the want of proper material to make nurses of was realised. The only way to obtain such was to improve the position, so that the work was limited and the conditions improved. Now there is a fairly numerous staff of probationers, of excellent quality on being trained [This was written four years after the school of nursing had opened]. Some old system day nurses were pensioned off, some joined the new system. Some could not change and left. The old night nurses, with careful watching and improved status, made good scrubbers and ward maids. All this was thanks to the zeal and energy of those ladies and nurses who began this work. The good effects are now seen in the high character of all the staff nurses. All nurses, night and day, are now of the same stuff and are carefully trained.

'The system of training is very complete. Probationers are first placed under the head nurse of the ward to learn the more mechanical part of the work, for though they have no menial duties to perform, it is thought well that they should know all that has to be done in a ward and know how to do it. They are then taught practical nursing and attend classes given by the lady superintendent. Then, with a practical and theoretical grounding, they attend lectures given by many of the medical officers of the Royal Infirmary, e.g. Mr Chiene on anatomy, Mr Croom on obstetrics and Mr Joseph Bell on surgical nursing and appliances. The emphasis is on practical nursing and on being able to help the doctors by giving correct reports on patients.

'Such a system cannot but produce good nurses to the comfort and well being of patients, both in the Infirmary and, it is hoped ere long, when the establishment is fully developed, of those of the wealthier classes whom sickness may compel to apply for help to the school of nursing in the Royal Infirmary.

'Above all there is now an esprit de corps, loyalty and self-respect, which has a most salutary effect on the whole tone of ward life, on patients and even on medical students. The coarseness, levity and hardness has been greatly modified and softened. The solitary meal, snatched at odd times in a nurse's room, is replaced by a meal eaten in a common hall, the cheerfulness and society of which must be a great rest.

'We need not speak here of the different class of society from which hospital nurses are now drawn. That many ladies by birth and breeding are now staff nurses is not a necessary part of the scheme, but it is a great advantage in many ways and we fearlessly assert that a lady, when inclination leads her to it, can be a probationer and nurse in a great hospital without the loss of her self-respect and without danger to her health. She can then lead a happy, useful and honourable life.

'It has been objected that the new system is expensive. It does cost money; everything from surgical dressings to horseflesh is dear nowadays, but, as a highly trained staff nurse with charge of, perhaps, thirty patients gets at most £25 per year, and a probationer £10, they can hardly be said to be overpaid. But were the expense double, no one who knows the difference the last twenty years has seen in our great hospital as to these matters, would grudge a shilling that has been spent in raising the status, character and career of that most valuable class, hospital nurses.'

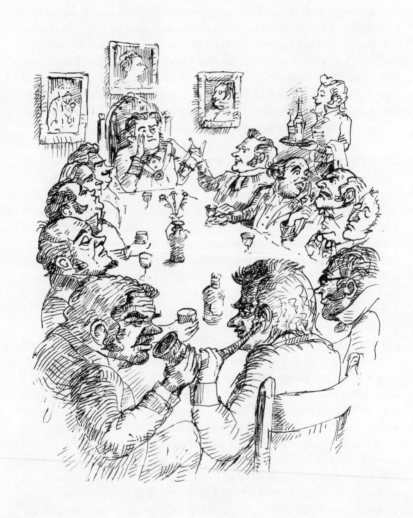

☙ 3 ☙

The Board of Management

I have never been able to conceive how any rational person could
propose happiness to himself from the exercise of power over others.

THOMAS JEFFERSON, *Writings*

Those who managed the Royal Infirmary of Edinburgh from 1840 to
1850 had every reason to go home after their monthly meeting very
well satisfied with their day's work. Their records show that they
were fair and considerate people. They could be generous but they
also appreciated financial savings, in such matters, for example, as the
numbers of leeches purchased from Mr Friedlander [see chapter 14].
They required staff and patients to conform to high standards of
behaviour. They ran, in other words, what the Royal Navy calls 'a
tight ship', a phrase usually followed by the encouraging maxim 'and
a tight ship is a happy ship!'

Other chapters deal with the Infirmary's logistical and financial
affairs, especially in the high-demand years of the 'fever' epidemics. In
the present chapter the rest of the work of the board is looked at
through extracts from the secretary's leather-bound minute books.
The topics discussed are both serious and trivial but the amusing
skirmishes with the younger doctors on the staff require a chapter to
themselves. The size of the management task the board faced can be
inferred from the annual number of admissions to the hospital. The
lowest annual total in the decade was 3,252, the highest 7,435.

The charter of the Infirmary required there to be twenty board
members, fourteen of whom had to be holders of public office. They
included the Lord Provost as chairman, the trade convener of the
Edinburgh city council, a number of representatives from the Colleges
of Surgeons and Physicians, a senator of the College of Justice, one
member of the Faculty of Advocates, one member of the Society of
Writers to the Signet (a solicitor) and one minister of the gospel. In

13

addition there were six 'contributors to the Infirmary' living in or near Edinburgh. The latter were not limited by occupation or other criteria. The following extracts show these people at work. It was unusual for all twenty members to be at any one meeting.

30 October 1840. Visiting Hours were to be 10–11 and 5–7. If a visitor was allowed to stay all night, no food was to be provided 'unless nursing duties were required'.

28 December 1842. McNab, the porter warned for drunkenness and neglect of duty. [He was later dismissed]

18 January 1841. Candidates for Edinburgh Royal Infirmary clerkships had to have passed their first exam for the medical degree in Edinburgh, or have a diploma from the Royal College of Surgeons of Edinburgh. This meant that students from England or elsewhere were excluded. This was now changed, applications being allowed if evidence of equal amounts of study could be provided.

8 March 1841. It was agreed that females should be searched at the outer gate by the wife of the porter and that she should receive an allowance of £5 per annum. [The reason for the search is not stated]

The Old Town dispensary requested the use of the recently installed vapour and hot baths at the Infirmary for their patients and would pay for this. This was agreed to as 'of much importance to the health of the lower orders'.

30 August 1841. Mr Christie, assistant apothecary, whose brief foray into nursing supervision is told in the section on 'nursing', was appointed house surgeon at Leith Hospital.

8 November 1841. It was suggested by Mr McKay that flannel dressing gowns should be allowed for the use of the patients in the wards at night.

On 15 May 1842 Professor Syme wrote to the board concerning the state of the surgical hospital where 'what writers in military surgery describe as hospital sore and hospital gangrene occur. The unequivocal effect of hospital air is to produce erysipelas, inflammation of the veins and inflammatory affections of the mucous membranes. These carry off a fearful number of the patients, so that recovery after serious operations and particularly amputations, has come to be regarded as a remarkable occurrence'.

It was resolved to tackle this by a series of measures. The surgical wards were to be moved to the empty fever hospital in Surgeons' Square. The wards were then to be fumigated and washed. Attention was to be paid to ventilation and drainage. None of the Surgeons' Square patients was to be returned to the Royal Infirmary's wards. No extra beds were to be put up in the wards. Bed spaces were to be clearly painted on the wall above the top of each bed, on which a 'ticket' was to bear the patient's name. Finally if money could be found, all male patients, after being put into the warm bath on admission, should be supplied with hospital dress consisting of serge gown, waistcoat and trousers with nightcap and carpet shoes and shirt if necessary. Their own clothes were to be laid aside until dismission. This would also save wear and tear on bedclothes, the men not lying down thereon in their own clothes. The bedding should be of straw and frequently destroyed and never reused after soiling. Finally the fever hospital was to be closed as quickly as possible [because of cost].

10 October 1842. Letters had been received from a series of leading London and other hospitals describing their policy and the views of their staff on mixing or segregating fever patients. The hospitals included Guy's and Bart's. Richard Bright wrote from Guy's. There was no concurrence among them.

1843 (early). Professor Syme was in trouble with the board following a complaint by the police about Mrs Malloy, wife of a scavenger, who had been brought to the Infirmary with burns. It was said that she had been refused admission to a general surgical ward on the grounds that such patients 'stank'. Her family was upset as they understood they would have to take her home. She was admitted to ward 10, the 'difficult case' ward, and Syme was said to have seen her only once in the eight days 'she languished on her death bed'. A manager had been responsible for getting her admitted to ward 10 and Syme claimed she was not his case. Fortunately Syme's clerk did visit and care for her. This case led to the board defining clinical responsibility of staff more clearly, and a special room for burns cases was opened.

Other surgeons complained to the board that Syme was giving all the surgery lectures, and that agreement about timing of lectures and operations could not be reached.

17 April 1843. Patients' diets were defined as low, common, full and extra. This, with a choice of bread or porridge for breakfast or supper, was claimed to represent eight diets. New items being added to the diets were tea at 4/6*d.* per lb., coffee (burnt) at 20*d,* essential oil of lemon at 1/6*d.* per oz. and eggs at 8*d.* per dozen new-laid, and at 4*d.* per dozen 'when preserved from Autumn in lime water or suet.'

Meals were breakfast, dinner and supper [but not for the clerks who had all the formal meals of the period]. Those ordering meals for patients were to stick to the eight diets without requesting changes, 'as this upset kitchen staff'. 'A 'full' diet was:

> Breakfast – 1½ pints of oatmeal porridge, butter, milk 1 pint.
> Dinner – Boiled meat 6 oz., potatoes 10 oz., and bread 3 oz., broth (barley, vegetables and meat)
> Supper – Potatoes 10 oz., new milk ½ pint.'

29 July 1844. With regard to these patients who have been upwards of two months in the hospital, who are incapable of further cure, and who therefore ought to be removed, the case of James Porteous in ward 6 was taken into consideration. The treasurer-superintendent was to get the history of Porteous and report to the next meeting.

12 July 1844. The papers of Porteous were sent to Mr Small, the treasurer of the Edinburgh charity workhouse, 'with a written re-quest that the patient might be immediately removed. This was agreed to and would be done that afternoon by the workhouse sending their own officers for him'.

At the same meeting the appointment of a resident clerk to the wards under the care of Mr Cormack was taken into consideration. The managers having considered the testimonials produced by A. F. Calder, John Struthers and Matthew Combe agreed to appoint Mr Struthers. 'The managers felt some difficulty in deciding this ap-pointment, each of the other gentlemen being very well qualified for the office from the high testimony borne to their professional attain-ments and character.'

20 July 1844. It was noted that the Cottage (No 9) which is kept for accidents by burning, is at present full of ordinary surgical cases and, of course, in the event of a burning accident occurring, there is no bed vacant. [This problem took a long time to sort out, no surgeon wanting to look after these cases]

5 May 1845. The director of the maternity hospital in the Canongate requested that 'part of the Royal Infirmary be set aside for puerperal fever cases when this epidemic might occur'.

At the same meeting it was noted that James Fortune, bandage maker to the Infirmary had died. William Richardson, a cutler, 'who offered bandages at a considerably lower price than did James's son Robert, and warranted them of equal quality', was appointed the new supplier.

26 May 1845. A letter was read from Captain Haining of the Police in which he complained about the 'detention' of two of his men at the Infirmary for twenty minutes, no surgeon coming after they had brought in a seriously injured patient. A letter of apology was sent

29 September 1845. Mr Edward Miller, who had been acting as a medical attendant in Jamaica, and who was to accompany Mr Waddell to west Africa on a missionary expedition, asked permission to attend the wards of the Infirmary for the two months he is to be in Edinburgh 'in order to improve the little practical acquaintance he has with disease and medicine'. The board gave him permission and agreed to 'remit the fees as he is not a regular medical student who intends applying for a diploma. He is not to interfere in any way with the treatment of cases'.

3 January 1846. Dr Thomson of York Place complained that the managers had 'connected a school of medicine with what he considered the proper use of the Infirmary, namely the treatment of the sick'. This was rejected as Thomson declined to make a formal motion of complaint. The Lord Provost, who was in the chair, took the opportunity to compliment the hospital on its work.

30 November 1846. A letter was read from the Royal Maternity Hospital, Milton House, Canongate.

26 November.

Puerperal fever having broken out in the Maternity Hospital we are under the necessity of shutting up the House for a time. There are at present five undelivered women whom it would be improper to have confined in the hospital and, not well knowing how to get the accòmmodation, we should feel very greatly obliged if your honourable board will favour us for a week or two with a ward in the fever hospital [i.e. in Surgeons' Square.]

17

This was agreed to but the arrangement was not eventually needed.

11 October 1847. David Cossar, son of the late Alex, the Infirmary's carpenter for many years, petitioned the board on behalf of his mother. He asked if they would give her money to buy a mangle for the support of herself and her family. On account of his father's faithful service, and 'he having died of fever caught in the performance of his duties', the board gave her £10.

The police asked the Infirmary to 'repair the Drummond Street pavement along the City Wall'. [Later the boundary wall at Carnegie Street also required attention]
A pauper now being defined simply as 'someone entitled to relief', the board were keen to get contributions from the inspectors of the poor.

27 Novemeber 1847. Dr McKellar, an extra physician, had died of fever. [One of many staff who died of fever, among them doctors old and young, nurses, at least one administrator, a porter and the hospital carpenter, Alex Cossar].
9 May 1848. The management of noisy patients was discussed. Causes included delirium tremens, and the delirium and impending delirium of fever. These patients were to be accommodated in ward 10, the 'seclusion ward'. Grouped with them were to be 'the dirty, for example those found lying in the street, or those who were suffering from unmanageable incontinence, especially where associated with the delirium stage of fever'.
6 October 1848. A special meeting. Two cases 'having all the symptoms of Asiatic cholera' had been admitted to ward 13' on the 5th October and both had died. They were Elizabeth Kinnear, aged 2, and John Kinnear, aged 12, from the West Port. Their father was a painter. Both had been ill for four days before admission. It was decided to use wards 7 and 17 as male and female cholera wards if more cholera cases came in. It was further decided 'to place at the disposal of the authorities, or as a board of Health acting under their orders [*sic*], the hospital in Surgeons' Square formerly used as a fever hospital, as well as a recently acquired nearby house (Dr Thomson's)'. These were to be furnished with beds and bedding. Nurses would be provided. After this, no more costs were to be laid at the board's door in administering relief to any cholera patients.

23 October 1848. Dumfries Hospital asked if cholera patients were to be admitted to Edinburgh Royal. This had not yet been finally decided. A letter was read from Kirknewton's Inspector of the Poor saying he has 'appropriated a house for the receiving of cholera cases if any should occur' and asking for the loan of two iron bedsteads. This was agreed.

Dr Christison wrote to the board suggesting that, instead of the open chair now used to convey cholera patients to the hospital, a palanquin, such as was used in the former epidemic of this disease be used. Instead of the patients arriving in a state of collapse they would, with a quantity of blankets and also bottles of hot water or hot sandbags, be kept in an advantageous state of warmth. This was agreed.

The Police asked for daily reports on the number of cholera cases and the districts affected. The authorities in Leith were told that, as Leith was too far away, it would be 'too damaging' for any cholera patients there to come to the Royal Infirmary. The city parochial board requested use of the Surgeons' Square hospital. This was agreed.

30 October 1848. A letter of thanks was received from city parochial board. As the parochial board was taking this initiative, the Infirmary now decided it would not admit cholera cases, sending them instead to this fever hospital.

2 November 1848. At this special meeting the parochial board of St Cuthbert's offered 9d. per patient per day if the Royal would take their cholera cases. They were told that the Royal had resolved not to take cholera patients. St Cuthbert's were thus left to send their cases to Surgeons' Square which they did not want to do as the city parochial board was to run it.

A letter was read from the staff surgeon, Edinburgh Castle, seeking right of admission for passed recruits billeted in the High Street, should the need arise. He also was told to send any patients to Surgeons' Square and pay the city parochial board.

Dr Martin Lamb resigned his clerk's post in the Infirmary having been appointed by the parochial board as resident medical officer to the cholera hospital (i.e. the Surgeons' Square hospital).

January 1849, Annual meeting. Regarding the large number of deaths in 1848, the board noted: 'This melancholy feature in the returns arises from no causes within the control of the managers or of their indefatigable medical and surgical officers.' Many who died were admitted terminally ill and a great majority of the patients, here and in Glasgow, was composed of the 'wandering Irish among whom the disease was much more prevalent and fatal than among the people of this country. Had they not been admitted, spread in the city would have been worse'. For some weeks also, the prevalence of influenza in the UK had led to deaths.

The board wished to prevent Edinburgh's exposure to 'Irish vagrants and paupers carrying pestilence in their wake' and would support 'any sanitary bill which may be introduced into Parliament . . .' At the end of this meeting the Lord Provost told members that he had just heard from the Lord Advocate that the latter was to introduce a Sanitary Bill for Scotland in Parliament this session. The meeting decided to appoint a committee to discuss the Bill with the Lord Advocate.

The city parochial board had opened convalescent houses for typhus victims during the year.

The high reputation of the Infirmary throughout all districts of Scotland and the north of England and improving transport had led to admissions from places from which people would not before have been removed.

The board agreed that a Royal Naval assistant surgeon be allowed to spend time attending the wards. Another attended later.

5 February 1848. A deputation from the city parochial board was seen and the Infirmary board agreed to take back control of the fever [now cholera] hospital in Surgeons' Square as cases were very much diminished. There had been no new ones for several days. The Infirmary managers agreed to look after the patients but would send the bill to the parochial board.

19 November 1848. The wards with brick floors, now worn, were to have them replaced with wood and stone pavement as in the principal medical wards.

And so, as the decade ended, there was relief that both the 'fever' and the cholera epidemics were almost over. The Royal Infirmary had coped well, living up to what it was now aware was its growing reputation.

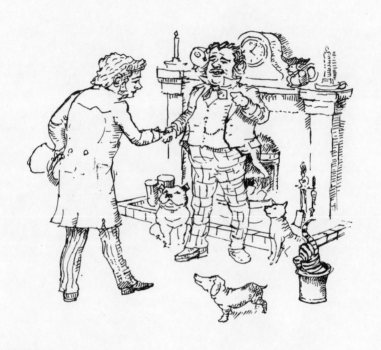

❧ 4 ❧

One of the Surgeons

Oh, Lord, it's hard to be humble . . .

POPULAR SONG

Robert Syme was one of Edinburgh's many famous professors of surgery. He held the post throughout the 1840s. Much has been written about him. The following notes come mostly from contemporary patients' records, the minutes of the Royal Infirmary's board of management, and editorials and correspondence in the *Lancet.*

It is true that Syme was one of the most able and conscientious surgeons of the pre-anaesthetic era. It is also true that he was one of the first European surgeons to use ether and then chloroform anaesthesia. In the 1860s he was quick to welcome the new antiseptic method of his assistant and son-in-law, Lister, having recorded his worries about post-operative infection at an earlier date. But he was a controversial figure with a prickliness of manner and an ability to generate powerful emotion in some who worked with him. Hamilton Bailey, an English surgeon of more modern times, described him as 'a genial happy man and a lover of flowers, whose contemporaries said of him that he never wasted a word, a drop of ink, or a drop of blood.' (Hamilton Bailey, *Notable Names in Medicine and Surgery,* H. K. Lewis, London, 1983) On the other hand, the degree to which he could raise hackles is seen in the following letter, written on the day of the event it describes and published in the *Lancet* on 23 February 1843:

> Sir – The uniformly uncourteous and uncivil demeanour of Professor Syme towards some parties in the wards of Edinburgh Royal Infirmary burst out so offensively against one of his clerks in that institute today, that I am at once prompted to ask you to notice it with a view to correct it, for it is alike unbecoming a professor and a gentleman. At the visit hour of twelve o'clock

today, as Mr Syme was examining a case of burns, he made some remark on the impropriety of applying cotton to burns, to which the clerk, Dr Andrews, replied in the most civil manner that the cotton was applied before the patient was admitted. The professor, as though he had been harbouring a feeling of animosity towards the clerk, broke out into a remarkable passion before patient and student, exclaiming 'Sir, it is no matter whether it was applied before or after admission, and I beg that you will trouble me with no more of your remarks!' The students of Edinburgh have for a number of years suffered from the uncourteous behaviour of Mr Syme and the sudden ebullitions of his temper and they, one and all, would be obliged by your mention of the undignified demeanour by which Mr Syme has so long been distinguished and the feeling which this has naturally created amongst them. I remain, Sir, an Edinburgh student.'

EDINBURGH'S 'MAYO CLINIC'

A row with his cousin Robert Liston meant that Syme had been refused a surgical job in the Royal in 1829. Typically he then opened his own private hospital in Minto House. This was a Mayo Clinic-type surgical hospital where he accommodated large numbers of surgical cases and taught pupils. His fame spread rapidly. In 1833, when Liston went to a chair in London, the University appointed Syme to the chair of clinical surgery and the Infirmary's board appointed him a junior assistant surgeon. They directed that 'with a view to maintaining the intimate connection between the Royal Infirmary and the University of Edinburgh, three wards containing thirty beds shall be put immediately under the charge of Professor Syme.' In this manner Syme added these prestigious appointments to the largest private practice in Scotland. His position at the top of Edinburgh's surgical pecking order could not have been more secure.

SYME AND THE *LANCET*

It is, therefore, disappointing that he went on to become so frequently involved in trivial disagreements. He might, for example, have avoided the unflattering interest of the *Lancet* on at least two other occasions in the 1840s. First he allowed a minor matter to get out of hand. The journal, in an editorial note of 16 May 1840, wrote:

Robertson v. Syme

The Edinburgh doctors are warring most spiritedly amongst themselves to the no small amusement of the more peaceable lookers-on. What is to become of the patients when the doctors' minds are engrossed with awful thoughts of legal perdition against their rivals? We have before us a letter addressed by Mr Syme to the Lord Provost, relating to an 'association of private lecturers calling themselves Queen's College'. Mr Syme it appears was anything but pleased with some of their remarks; the lawyers were consulted and the case very nearly merged into the title which we have selected for the heading of this paragraph.

Again, on 27 February 1841, the *Lancet* published a letter from a 'medical observer' commenting on an article by Syme in the *Edinburgh Monthly Journal of Medical Science*. It was headed 'Mr Syme and the Edinburgh Surgeons' and begins:

Mr Syme lists seven operations he has done, with success, for popliteal aneurysm, involving the tying of the femoral artery. 'In the same time', Syme goes on, 'four done by others had ended unfavourably.' 'These other surgeons', the writer notes unsurprisingly, 'took exception to this', especially when Syme continued, 'While it is usual to attribute untoward occurrences [in surgery] to the patient, I am quite sure that attention to some minor points in performing the operation has a much larger share in determining a favourable outcome.'

This was certainly confrontational and provoked retaliation. In their reply Syme's fellow surgeons quoted lithotomy statistics. 'These' they said, 'give an idea of Mr Syme's surgical skill far from favourable. In lithotomy, and in general surgery, Syme's surgical skill is much inferior to that of Mr Robertson. To be second to Robertson is, however, no disparagement to Syme or to any surgeon.' They conclude their letter by saying, 'Syme should not do these numerical comparisons, as they engender professional dislikes which have so long been the disgrace of medical men.' [This book contains a description of an operation on a femoral aneurysm carried out by Syme in 1841]

Syme went to London briefly in 1847 on Liston's death, having been elected to the latter's post in University College Hospital. He did not like the atmosphere and returned to Edinburgh in a few months to take up all his old appointments. This unusual event once again caught the *Lancet*'s eye. Its sarcastic comments are quoted in this book in the section on 'Edinburgh and the Medical Press'.

SYME AND THE BOARD OF MANAGEMENT

The Royal Infirmary's board of management throughout this decade had frequent difficulties with their senior surgeon. In 1840, for example, he was in dispute with the managers about the number of senior surgeons on the Infirmary staff, claiming that his access to appropriate 'teaching' cases was being restricted.

His longest running battle with them, however, was over his refusal to sign his clerks' weekly ward journals. The board of management had decided that it must see every ward's journal every week, each journal to be counter-signed before submission by the ward's physician or surgeon in charge. A clerk's duties included the keeping of this journal, which contained details of each patient's history and progress, the treatment given and a discharge summary. [These are the journals which provide the case histories quoted in this book]. The board checked the journals and recorded the checks in their minutes. All the Infirmary's physicians and surgeons complied with this requirement except Syme, who considered the check unnecessary. A number of the journals from various wards have survived. Only Syme's are unsigned.

His refusal to sign was a breach of the board's ruling and it now became a matter of prestige. Many attempts to persuade Syme failed and finally he was told that he was to be dismissed from his Infirmary post. His University job was not at risk, being under a different authority, but the situation nearly arose in which the University's professor of clinical surgery would have been barred from the surgical wards of the Infirmary. This was too much, even for Syme. Christison found him a way out, which is not absolutely clear, but which included making the award of a clerk's final certificate dependent on his chief signing a book monthly, to say he was doing a good job. Syme agreed grudgingly. From his home in Charlotte Square he wrote to the board:

> Gentlemen . . . I now acquaint you of my intention of complying with the instruction. At the same time I take the liberty of

expressing my deep regret at being forced to perform a duty which will every week prevent me from forgetting how little respect for my opinions as to the professional details of the hospital is entertained by the managers and how lightly they value my connection with the Infirmary.'

IN THE OPERATING THEATRE

When operating, Syme was even more able to make his presence felt. On one occasion he complained, probably quite fairly, of noise in the theatre. The managers at once ordered that 'A board is to be put up reading "The managers desire that complete silence be maintained in the theatre during the whole time of the performance of operations".'

Twenty-two students wrote to the board in June 1845 complaining 'that Professor Syme was in the practice of performing important operations in the presence of his own class to the exclusion of all other students'. Syme's reply to this was swift and cooperative. The board noted at their next meeting that 'Mr Syme agrees to conform to Regulations and all students will now be able to witness the performance of capital or important operations, or, as designated by the late Professor Charles Bell, 'the great operations of surgery namely trepan, hernia, amputation, aneurism and lithotomy', besides others well known in surgery'.'

His students would have appreciated the range of Syme's skill when he operated on Mary Blackwell. There was no specialist ENT surgeon in Edinburgh Royal until 1883. Syme had an audience in theatre when he carried out a tricky procedure which is made to sound simple in his clerk's report:

MARY BLACKWELL, aged 53
Kinghorn, Fife. Husband a factory man.
25 July 1848. Admitted to surgical wards of Professor Syme. Three years ago she had a large nasal polypus removed which pointed backwards and hung down into the pharynx. She continued until eighteen months ago when her old symptoms began to return, consisting chiefly of a constant feeling of stuffiness of the nose and latterly of a difficulty of breathing and a sensation of choking.

On examination by the mouth, a large excrescence is found protruding beyond the soft palate and uvula.

Mr Syme, in the presence of the class, introduced a pair of polypus forceps by the anterior nares and, having destroyed the attachment of the polypus, the woman spat out an enormous mass having the usual consistence of such tumours.

29 July 1848. Dismissed cured.

'SYME'S AMPUTATION'

In 1844 Syme reported a series of fourteen cases of foot injury requiring amputation. The operation he preferred involved removal of the foot through the ankle joint. With mobilisation of wide flaps this had the advantage of allowing weight to be borne subsequently on tissue already adapted for that purpose. The operation became known as 'Syme's amputation' and was in use for many years after his death in 1870. The difficulty of fitting a suitable prosthesis, however, eventually led to it being abandoned.

AND fiNALLY . . .

Finally a typical anecdote to finish these brief notes on a brilliant but difficult man. Syme worked for many years with James Young Simpson, and made full use of chloroform when it replaced ether. He did not, however, remain on good terms with his now equally famous colleague. Their relationship ended on an unhappy note. Simpson had been ill and when eventually he realised he was dying he went to see Syme and held out his hand to say goodbye. But Syme was as unyielding as ever. Standing with his back to the fire he took Simpson's hand and said 'You have come to apologise, have you?'

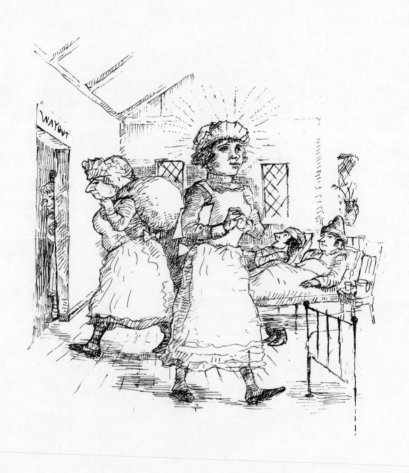

❦ 5 ❦

Two Matrons

Hath not the potter power over the clay, of the
same lump to make one vessel unto honour, and
another unto dishonour?

Romans 9:20

The Infirmary had two matrons in the 1840s. One served the hospital
well; the other did not. At that time a hospital matron had different
responsibilities from those she had in more modern times. She was
less involved with the nursing staff and more concerned with
management of the House, as the hospital was called, and the well-
being of the patients. Only when nursing became more clearly defined
as a profession, did she have to deal with both aspects equally. Now, of
course, she has gone for ever.

MRS WOOD

Mrs Wood from Dublin was appointed matron in 1840 from 'a very
numerous list of applicants'. She took up the post on the understanding that she had no responsibilities outside her duties. That
meant responsibilities to relatives, as an Edinburgh Royal matron at
that time was required to be single, or widowed without dependants,
'so that she would be divested of every other care but that of the
hospital, whose inmates she was to regard as her family'. It was,
therefore, a surprise for Mr McKay, an Infirmary board member, to
find on a routine hospital inspection eight months after Mrs Wood's
arrival, that, living in Mrs Wood's quarters were her daughter, her
daughter's baby and her daughter's servant. Mrs Wood had, moreover, appointed her daughter, Mrs Fleming, to be assistant matron of
the Royal Infirmary although, in fairness, she may have had the
authority to do so.

Matron's explanation was that Mr Fleming, her daughter's husband,
had died after she, Mrs Wood, had been appointed to Edinburgh Royal.

31

It was decided to let the arrangement continue 'at the pleasure of the board and in this case only; a regular charge to be made against Mrs Wood for the expense of Mrs Fleming's child and servant'.

Not much is known of the good side of Mrs Wood. With Dr Reid, the resident superintendent, she instigated the much-needed review of night nurse supervision. It was she also who arranged that 'convalescent patients would dine together, instead of in bed, this for the comfort of the patients and the cleanliness of the wards'.

But on 5 December 1842 Mrs Wood and her daughter were abruptly dismissed for dishonesty. The board's minutes record that the charges against them were that:

1   An oak chest of drawers and a glazed bookcase had been unlawfully removed from the Infirmary.
2   Four dish covers, bought from Sibbald's for Infirmary use, charged in his account against the hospital and certified by Mrs Wood as correctly charged, had in a similar way been sent away from the House by her, without ever having been employed therein.
3   The hospital wright had been much employed by Mrs Wood in making articles of hospital furniture for her own behoof.

The board had 'less hesitation in reaching the decision [to sack Mrs Wood] as she had requested leave to resign'. Mrs Fleming, however, wrote refuting the charges and saying her accusers should look at the cash books. This ploy backfired when board member Mr William Lizars, from the family optical firm which still flourishes in Edinburgh today, did just that. He testified to the board that one entry in the cash book was newer than those around it, and that another was in different ink. Mrs Wood's last throw was to write to the board saying that she was probably dying! She hoped, therefore, that for the sake of her family, no big fuss would be made.

This was a little optimistic, as Mrs Wood's brothers had also been removing 'unwanted' wood from the wright's shop. Three servants were dismissed at the same time, having been implicated in these activities. Less clear was the finding that one 'E. Walsh', described as a 'passage washer' and on the payroll, was in fact Mrs Fleming's maid, to whom no duties had been allocated in the Infirmary. Finally, it is recorded without comment in the same minutes that 'there had been no servant in the hospital of late of the name of Robertson,' and that 'there had been no sole employee as sempstress for a long time'.

The board of management, as on many occasions in the 1840s, acted leniently. No prosecution was brought but the items removed had to be returned.

MISS PEAT

Miss Peat was as honest as her predecessor was not. On 13 February 1843 she succeeded Mrs Wood as matron, the board noting with relief 'that she had no Edinburgh connection and no local friends or dependants to put temptation in her way'. She was not long, however, in finding troubles of her own. These were mainly with a series of unruly junior doctors for whose accommodation and food she as Matron was responsible.

First she weathered Dr Maitland's complaint that she had called him 'an inefficient clerk'. The board decided that he was more at fault than she in that he had left his ward when feeling ill. 'We consider that Dr Maitland acted rashly in deserting the important duties committed to him by Dr Dickson. We have received a statement from the Matron in which she denies having used any expression to Dr Maitland he could find consistent with her having called him "an inefficient clerk". She did not recollect his giving her a statement of ill health he had obtained from Dr Craigie but, on going to her room and searching for it, she found it. She thereupon returned to Dr Maitland's room and simply asked if this was the certificate to which he had alluded. We feel that there is no ground for the complaint against the Matron and that Dr Maitland should not, in any circumstances, have deserted the charge committed to him.'

Then she was in trouble for being too good to her charges! She was 'directed to act according to Hospital Regulations and provide only breakfast, dinner and tea for clerks, all luncheons and suppers to be discontinued, though any of the gentlemen may obtain biscuit or bread in the forenoon in the dining room'.

By October 1844 her kind-heartedness was wearing thin. She reported as follows. 'The hours for breakfast are very irregularly kept up by the clerks. This morning five gentlemen of the establishment were at breakfast till 10.20. This has occurred so frequently of late that the waiter now declines to remove the breakfast from before the gentlemen at 10 o'clock, as was ordered by the house committee. Some of the gentlemen had only then sat down to the meal. The serving man's time was required for other important duties within the hospital.' The board sent a letter to the clerks.

Shortly afterwards, the clerks sought Miss Peat out again, stating that 'they would consider it a great convenience if they were allowed to have their bread and milk or porridge at night placed in their rooms instead of their being obliged to come to the dining room'. As matron offered no objection, the managers agreed to this change being made, 'on the understanding that the bread and milk be placed in the clerks' rooms by the male attendant and that the arrangement is interim and by way of experiment'.

It was a rule of the Infirmary that senior members of its in-house staff dined with the resident doctors. In 1849 Miss Peat's difficulties with the doctors came to a head. She submitted a special report on their meal-time behaviour to the managers. This read as follows:

> The Matron complained that the clerks had treated her so as to prevent her joining them, as duty required, at the dinner table. They had destroyed articles of household use in a wanton manner and also articles of food set before them. This she knew was due to their dissatisfaction at the food and their accommodation. She disagreed with this and submitted a diet roll of lunch and dinner for the past six months, saying it was all right for her. She allowed that occasionally they might be right, the cooking not always being too good as cooks were hard to get, their hours and pay being unpopular.

The committee was surprised that she had not eaten with the clerks since 10 December last, and they interviewed the treasurer-superintendent, the chaplain, three clerks and the manservant or porter who waits at table. They found that:

1 The clerks were generally dissatisfied with their treatment in the hospital.
2 Matron had given up eating with them for their use of 'improper language' on one occasion, on top of the general treatment she got from them.
3 The treasurer-superintendent, 'partly for want of time, as he states', and partly from the disagreeable situation in which matters stood with the clerks, also ceased to dine with them.
4 The Chaplain stayed at the table but occasionally had to leave

in consequence of their behaviour. He always returned, either
at their request or because he thought he should.

5 This was inexcusable conduct from young men in such a
position.

6 The excuses of the clerks were not well founded.

It was resolved that the treasurer-superintendent was to return
to the table but that the matron need not, as yet. The committee
felt that 'the presence of a single woman such as matron at the
table is of no real benefit, and leaves her too open to inconsiderate
remarks. But the treasurer-superintendent or the chaplain must
again preside at the table and should not have stopped doing so.
While the clerks are open to censure they had indeed complained
of the food at a lower level and were reluctant to do so higher up.'

    The chairman finished by saying that, without agreeing whole-
heartedly with the clerks, the board would look at what they
could do to help. The clerks were called in and admonished.
Matron agreed to resume her place later.

  While the minutes contain nothing except favourable references to
this matron it does appear likely that she would have looked forward
to her days off!

UNUSUAL CASES FROM THE JOURNALS: I

SARAH GRAHAM, aged 20
Outworker
7 May 18??. Admitted to Ward 2. In good health until ten days ago. At that time an eruption appeared on her right side which she says began in the form of blisters which appeared gradually for five days and then peeled off. She worked during the first five days, her only complaint being a stitch at the lower right side. During the other five days she had no employment and she has had little food for some time.

On examination appears healthy. A band of eruption about two inches broad extends round the right side below the mamma from the spine to the sternum. There is none on the left side. It is of a red colour with minute scabs said to have been vesicles.
Applic: unguen: simplex [1]
10 May 18??. Pain and tenderness of epigastrium. Pulse natural but easily excited.
14 May 18??. Dismissed cured.
Diagnosis in ward journal – shingles

WILLIAM TAYLOR, aged 17
Warriston Close. A printer.
17 June 1844. Admitted to Surgical Wards of Professor Syme.

On the morning of the 14th he accidentally upset a cup filled with strong sulphuric acid. The contents fell upon his left leg and, before his trousers could be pulled off, a considerable injury was done to the skin.

On examination the course of the acid is marked by dark streaks consisting of superficial sloughs. The largest of these is over the inner side of the leg and a number of small ones are on the outer and anterior surfaces.

A poultice to be applied.
22 June 1844. Blue wash to be applied. [2]
22 July 1844. Dismissed cured.

---

[1] Apply simple ointment (made from white wax, prepared lard and almond oil)
[2] Blue Wash was probably a solution of copper sulphate.

ALEXANDER PRENTICE, aged 17
From County Antrim. A labourer.
5 September 1844. Admitted to surgical wards of Professor Syme.

On Monday the second September, when he was engaged in reaping, his left arm was stung, he thinks by a nettle. In the course of that day it became red, swollen and painful and has continued in that condition ever since.

On examination the whole of the forearm is found hot, red and swollen. Two fluctuating points are perceived above the wrist and on the outer side of the forearm.

These were opened immediately after admission.
16 September 1844. Dismissed cured.

DONALD CAMERON, aged 61
From Crieff parish. A gamekeeper.
27 May 1841. Admitted to surgical wards of Prof. Syme.

Admitted on account of a cancerous affection of the lower lip, close to the left angle of the mouth. Eight months ago a small portion was excised on account of a similar growth. Some induration remained and has since increased. At present the induration extends round the angle of the mouth for about three-quarters of an inch, chiefly towards the lower part. It is the seat of occasional lancinating pain which shoots down towards the angle of the jaw. Immediately below the base of the jaw, about its middle, an enlarged gland exists, hard and about the size of a bean. He has been in the constant habit of smoking tobacco for about thirty years.[1]
1 June 1841. The growth was today removed by a double incision above and below the tumour. The bleeding was stopped by torsion and one ligature was applied. Edges of the wound brought together by three interrupted sutures.
3 June 1841. Wound united in the whole extent.
5 June 1841. Stitches removed. Wound entirely healed.
15 June 1841. Dismissed cured.   R. M.

[1] Although not stated here, cancer of the lower lip was sometimes seen in those who had smoked clay pipes over a long period

MRS CLARK, aged 40
Works in fields. From Endrick parish.
19 June 1841. Admitted to Surgical Wards of Professor Syme.

About six months ago she first felt sharp pains in the right breast and on examination she discovered a small hard tumour the size of a pea about an inch below the nipple. Since that time the tumour has increased gradually, but more rapidly during the last two months.

It is now about the size of a bantam's egg, hard, partially adherent to the skin and situated a little below and to the inner side of the nipple. The breast has a natural appearance and the glands of the axilla are unaffected. The origin of the disease can be referred to no external circumstance. Her catamenia[1] continue and are regular in their appearance.

23 June 1841. The mamma was today excised in the usual manner. Profuse bleeding took place and ten vessels required ligature. Edges brought together by stitches and cold applied.

24 June 1841. Some bleeding took place during the afternoon which was repressed by the application of cold. The edges were approximated by adhesive straps and the cold continued. Today she is doing well but the breast appears distended by coagulum.

28 June 1841. The coagulum of blood has been nearly all discharged and healthy suppuration is going on. Edges retained in apposition with adhesive straps. Water dressing applied.

12 July 1841. Discharge greatly diminished. The extremities of the incision have united and the rest of the wound is cicatrising rapidly.

29 July 1841. Dismissed cured.

MATTHEW O'SHEA, aged 35
Uphall, formerly Donegal. A labourer.
23 May 1841. Admitted to Surgical Wards of Professor Syme. Five days ago his left hand was crushed in a crane. The tip of the forefinger was denuded of soft parts and the first [*sic*] phalanx was removed by a surgeon. Adhesive plaster was applied to the

---

[1] 'Catamenia' is an old word for menstrual periods.

wounds. On admission the finger was found gangrenous as far as the second phalanx where the line of demarcation was defined.

24 May 1841. Forefinger removed at MC articulation by making a flap from each side. Two vessels were tied. A wound exists on the fore and back parts of the middle finger to which a poultice was applied. The second phalanx is fractured. Feverishness present.

25 May 1841. Continues feverish. A good deal of redness around the wound and over greater part of hand. Antimonials given and a warm water dressing applied.

26 May 1841. During the night complained of pain in the back of the neck and of stiffness of the jaw and cold sweating. Skin cold and covered with perspiration. Jaw perfectly closed and fixed. Muscles behind shoulder and back of neck are stiff and painful. His countenance is pale and sunk; his expression is one of great anxiety. Stitches removed and a poultice applied to whole hand.

℞ *Fol. Nicot. Tabac.* 1 drachm.

Aqua tepid 16 oz.

Fiat infusum cujus sumat 1 drachm *quaq. hora.*[1]

27 May 1841. All the symptoms have increased since yesterday's report. The tobacco is continued. He is now unable to swallow. The muscles of the neck and jaw are perfectly rigid. He has frequent attacks of opisthotonus with twisting of the chest to the left. Unable to expectorate the mucus in the trachea and bronchi. Face livid.

27 May 1841. (later) He has had three attacks of convulsions, one at 6 am, one a little before noon and the last at 1 p.m. from which he did not recover. He was partially sensible till within two hours of death.   R. McKenzie

Diagnosis in ward register – amputations, tetanus.[2]

---

[1] The instruction is 'Make an infusion of which one drachm to be taken every hour.' Tobacco, as an infusion of Virginian tobacco leaves, was used according to Beasley, 'as an antispasmodic to relax the muscular system.'

[2] A post-mortem was carried out. 'The brain, spinal cord and membranes were carefully examined but no trace of morbid action was detected. The nerves in the region of the amputated finger were unaltered. The nerves of the middle finger were engaged in the laceration of the soft parts and the digital nerve on the ulnar side was found in an abscess cavity.' [This account implies that the aetiology of tetanus was unknown in 1841.]

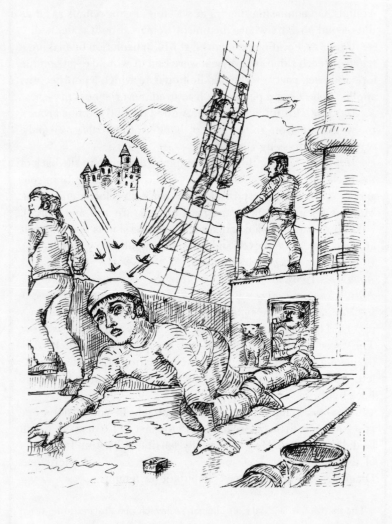

🎔 6 🎔

Ague

They told me I was every thing; 'tis a lie, I am not ague-proof.

SHAKESPEARE, *King Lear*

Edinburgh was ague-proof by the 1840s in that the disease, now better known as malaria, could not then be acquired in Scotland. It had, according to one source, been common in some districts of the country as late as 1800. It had certainly existed in England, as far north as Cambridgeshire, until early in the reign of Victoria. In the 1840, as the seamen in this chapter found, it could still be acquired remarkably far north in Europe.

Dr Christison, a physician at the Infirmary, describes how in 1827 he saw his first case of malaria. He called it 'intermittent fever' or 'tertian ague'. His patient was 'a reaper, harvesting in the Lincoln-shire fens', who went home to Kelso for treatment. The doctor there, however, had not seen a case. This was an indication of the decline of the disease in that area, the records of Kelso's dispensary showing that, around 1780, 70-160 cases of 'ague' were treated there annually. The Kelso man was referred to Edinburgh Royal Infirmary. Christison remembered him in his autobiography: 'I saw him in the waiting room having a violent rigor. He was admitted and given 18 grains of Sulphate of Quinia before the subsequent fit that was due. But he had no other, and went home well soon after.' Christison goes on 'I have treated since fifteen or sixteen cases of ague from Lincoln-shire, Cambridgeshire, the West Indies and India. My policy is to allow them to take one fit after admission before giving quinia.' This seems a canny way of confirming the diagnosis when only clinical methods are available.

By 1840 most of Edinburgh Royal Infirmary's cases came through the city's port of Leith. While seamen formed the majority, the records of ward 11 also recount the case of a woman who had just returned from the New World. The case notes of Joan McArthur and two seamen are reproduced below. The third seaman's case history is included as a curiosity.

JOAN MCARTHUR, aged 22
Perth. A domestic servant.
24 April 1849. Admitted to Edinburgh Royal Infirmary. States that her health has always been indifferent. Thirteen years ago had acute rheumatism. Twelve months back went to Greenwood, near New York, a place which she states 'is very malarious and where ague is prevalent [*sic*]'. She resided there three months and suffered from the heat and 'bad air'. Two days after being on board ship returning home was seized with shiverings followed by fever and profuse perspiration. These returned every other day for a week, after that occurring every day for six weeks. Had no medicine during that time but on her arrival at Perth took quinine and was cured.

Enjoyed tolerable health afterwards till one month ago when she suffered from indigestion. Four days before admission, that is on 21 April, was seized with a return of the rigors, which recurred again two days before admission.
25 April 1849. On admission expected to have a paroxysm which however did not occur. Some pain in head and back. On examining the region of the spleen dullness is heard over a considerable area.
27 April 1849. Has had no fit since admission.
30 April 1849. Dismissed by desire.

MALCOLM GREENSHIELDS, aged 16
Leith. A seaman.
19 June 1847. Admitted ward 11. Returned from Riga on Tuesday last at which place he states that he was first seized with the symptoms of ague five weeks ago. Says the disease was very prevalent among the sailors at that port. He never slept ashore during the night and he was the only person on the vessel who was affected.

At first the paroxysms were very severe but latterly much less so. The shivering fit comes on regularly about twelve o'clock midday and continues for about one hour, the hot stage for half an hour and the shivering stage for one and a half hours. From the frequent recurrence of the attacks he was much debilitated.

---

21 *June 1847*. Pulse has been steadily frequent and skin warm since admission. Skin moist at present. Some headache.

Hab: Pulv: Effervesc. [dose illegible] *qq hora..*[1]

23 *July 1847*. Dismissed cured.

Index of ward journal gives diagnosis as – intermittent fever-? malaria

JACK SHAW, aged unknown
From North Leith. A seaman.

13 July 1849 Admitted to ward 11. About six weeks ago, while engaged in cleaning out the vessel in which he was employed at Elsinore in Denmark, he slept on deck, after which exertion led to rigors. Recurring fits of rigors, sweating and weakness continued for twenty days and then every third day until admission.

14 *July 1849* At 1 pm had a rigor after which sweated. In evening felt pretty well.

℞ *Sulph: Bebeer:* grains 10 *hora somni, et cras.*[2]

15 *July 1849* To have 20 grains bebeerine before breakfast tomorrow and 20 grains at twelve o'clock.

16 *July 1849* Has had no regular fit of rigor but about the usual period of attack felt chilly.

Repet: Sulph: Bebeer: ut antea.[3]

18 *July 1849* No fit but feeling of coldness.

25 *July 1849* The bebeerine having been remitted, the attack has recurred as previous to admission.

℞ *Sulph: Quina:* grains 8. *Sumat* 1 *t.i.d. Talis 3*

℞ *Sulph: Quina:* grains 12. *Take tomorrow at twelve o'clock.*[4]

28 *July 1849* Has not suffered from the disease since the start of quinine. Dismissed at his own desire.   A. Christison[1]

Diagnosis in ward journal – ague

[1] To have an effervescent powder '*quaqua hora*' (every hour).

[2] Bebeerine is an alkaloid derived from the bark of the nectandra or Bebeeru tree. Used as the sulphate. A 'febrifuge'. Beasley lists four preparations of the drug, of which three are from Edinburgh doctors, one from W. T. Gairdner and two from Prof. R. Christison. The instruction here means 'to have 10 grains at bedtime, and tomorrow'.

[3] 'Repeat as formerly'.

[4] The first quinine prescription was to be repeated three times only ('*talis* means 'such a one.') The second was a 'once only' dose.

[5] Son of the professor.

FRANCIS FERGUSON, aged 59
Prestonpans, near Edinburgh. A seaman.
5 July 1847 Admitted to ward 11. About thirty years ago had an attack of ague which lasted for four months. Twelve years ago suffered from Coast Fever in Africa from which he recovered in fourteen days. Neither left any bad effect. Three months ago observed a swelling in the left hypochondrium and epigastrium, accompanied by a dragging pain on the left side of the chest aggravated by lying on the right side. During his last voyage was ashore two or three nights in Tunis. During the three days spent there, the ship lying near the shore, he was ashore several times in the day in the discharge of his duties. Was also ashore often at Malta. He attributes his complaint to something he ate or drank in Tunis.[1]
21 August 1847 Dismissed relieved.
19 October 1847. Readmitted. After leaving hospital he went to Prestonpans for the benefit of the sea air. But from the occurrence of easterly winds all his symptoms returned in aggravated style. On examination there was no change in size of the spleen from last admission.
30 November 1847. Dismissed by desire.
Diagnosis in ward journal – disease of spleen.

[1] Coast fever, possibly also known as Gambia fever, could have been one of many diseases. One source states that Gambia fever was caused by trypanosoma gambiense. In this, as in other tropical illness, the spleen may be enlarged.

THEORIES ABOUT AGUE

There was great puzzlement at this time about the cause of the disease. The word malaria was formed from 'mal-aria' or 'bad air.' When, for example, a Mrs Barker was admitted to the Royal Infirmary in 1846, with a pyrexia of unknown origin, it was thought worthy of note that 'she had never had ague or been in any miasmic district.' The word 'miasma' crops up frequently in these early records, describing the damp, misty atmosphere around the marshy areas in which the disease was found. The fact that such conditions also favour the breeding of mosquitoes was probably noticed but its significance was not appreciated.

Christison referred again to disease-producing miasmas when, also in 1846, he published a paper in the *Edinburgh Medical Journal* on an unrelated disease. This was 'An account of a typhoid fever apparently originating in a local miasma'. The title demonstrates another contemporary confusion in its misleading adjectival use of the word 'typhoid'. This is discussed in the chapter on the fever epidemics.

Many theories were put forward, among them that of Dr Henry McLeish of Belfast contained in his letter to the *Edinburgh Medical Journal* of 25 May 1843. His belief was 'that the poisonous impregnation of the atmosphere termed 'malaria' or 'marsh miasma' is in every case, of vegetable origin'. He wrote:

> I do not agree with Ferguson in your last number, as I do not think that malaria is an emanation from the elemental soil. My assertion is that in every case it is of vegetable origin. The Sahara is as free from the disease as is the ocean itself because in the one there is heat but no moisture and no vegetation; in the other warmth and moisture enow but of vegetation none. Quit the murderous coast of Africa for the desert or the ocean and you are free from the murderous malaria, in a word totally exempt from the source of the disease. And yet there is an exception in the case of the sea which fortunately is conclusive of the question. Vessels have left a malarious shore still free from periodic disease; perchance they have never even touched at a malarious spot; but after they have been a certain time under the burning sun the vegetable filth which sometimes collects on board in the many corners and crannies of a ship gives out fatal poison. The result is the well proved production of remittent yellow fever [*sic*], in the lower decks especially, as much as in the midst of the most infected marsh or otherwise malarious locality.

It took another fifty years for anopheline mosquitoes to be confirmed as the vectors of malaria. A Scot, Ronald Ross, made the discovery in August 1897. He dissected a mosquito which had fed on a man suffering from malaria and found in its gut the protozoon *Plasmodium.* This was known to be present in other humans with the disease. The discovery won Ross a Nobel Prize in 1902.

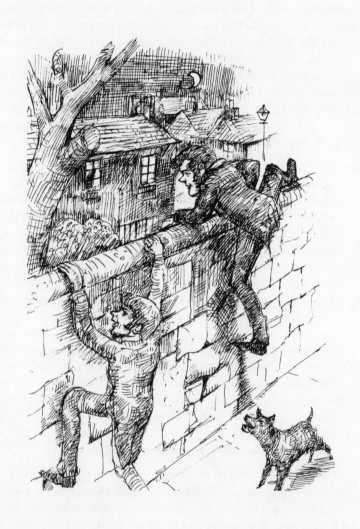

7

Controlling the Junior Doctors

Gin by pailfuls, wine in rivers,
Dash the window glass to shivers!
For three wild lads were we, brave boys,
And three wild lads were we.

SCOTT, *Guy Mannering*

Sir Walter's wild lads were no wilder than the young doctors of the Royal Infirmary in the 1840s. The latter would no doubt have claimed that they were simply following in the footsteps of their predecessors. John Reid, for example, when a medical student in 1826 took part 'for love of adventure, in the affrays which followed grave-robbing by rival bands'. This astonished the more staid Robert Christison with whom he shared lodgings. Christison, later to be a senior physician in the Infirmary, was equally horrified when he realised that his junior colleague Mowbray Thomson was in the habit of climbing out of the Royal Infirmary at night to join the later resurrectionists, 'as he said "for adventure!" '

To graduate MD in Edinburgh a student had to complete four years of study and be twenty-one years old. He had to pass the examinations set by the University, be competent in Latin and have a dissertation examined. In 1841 the MD was conferred on one hundred and three men who had 'gone through the appropriate examinations and defended publicly their Inaugural Dissertations'. So many 'overseas' graduates with British names are listed in the 1840s that some must have been the sons of Empire-building expatriates. Graduates in that year came from Scotland, England, Ireland, Gibraltar, Nova Scotia, New Brunswick, Canada, North America, Jamaica, St Vincent, Barbadoes [*sic*], Ceylon, East Indies, Italy and Poland. In 1843 they came, in addition, from Buenos Aires, Genoa, St Helena, Bermuda, Brazil and Antigua.

There were opportunities for the new doctors to work as 'dressers' in the Infirmary's wards and there was much competition for the six posts of resident 'clerk'. These were the 'house doctors' of today. The most formal part of a clerk's day was the visit of the senior doctor, in charge of the ward. He arrived 'at certain and specific times'. The clerk then had to read aloud his reports on the patients, providing information on 'Date, bed, operation of medicine, intervening symptoms, pulse, urine, faeces, spittle, tongue, thirst, appetite, ordinary symptoms, supernumerary symptoms, food, drink and medicine'. The senior doctor 'then dictated to the clerk his views of the condition, with comments and prescription'. These ward rounds did not always proceed smoothly, as the section on Professor Syme in this book shows.

The clerks worked long hours and were often in trouble with the board of management. The following extracts from the board minutes shed light on the activities of these young men and their reasonably tolerant elders.

17 February 1840. Clerks reprimanded for ordering tobacco for their patients from the Apothecary's shop. The wards were non-smoking.

11 October 1841. It was noted that a letter had appeared in 'The Scotsman' of last Wednesday stating that a patient had waited one hour in the Surgical Hospital suffering from an accident without receiving any attention and had then left the hospital to seek it elsewhere. The board reprimanded the clerks.

20 May 1844. Dr Kelburne King came in at 2.15 and was warned of dismissal.

8 July 1844. Dr Kelburne King absent all night on 6 July [but got away with a reprimand].

14 August 1844. An Extraordinary meeting of the board was convened to consider why Dr Fleming, the clerk, had not been in attendance when he ought to have been on the arrival of a seriously injured man. The man, from Donaldson's Institution, had a fracture of the thigh. A proper deputy, i.e. one of the other resident clerks, had not been substituted and the patient was dealt with by Mr Howieson, an assistant to the Apothecary, assisted by a nurse. Howieson 'had to do the important operation of reducing the fracture and setting the limb. It was, however, well done'.

Dr Fleming was called in and, having been heard in explanation, the managers decided that Dr Fleming's grounds for leaving the patients under his care were quite untenable. He was told by the chairman 'that a Resident clerk should have been substituted, that he was to be more on his guard in the future, that he was to bestow all due care on the patients entrusted to him and was to obey the regulations for resident clerks in all respects'.

19 August 1844. The managers had seen the time book from which it appeared that Dr Shand, a resident clerk, was absent on the evening of the 13th inst and till one o'clock of the following morning. That on the evening of the 17th he was absent in like manner and remained out till one in the morning and that on the 18th he was likewise out till midnight, and that he had obtained leave to be out, by writing to the Superintendent, on only one of those occasions.

The time book also showed that on 16th May last Dr John Shand came in at one twenty in the morning and that he was warned thereafter that dismissal would follow unless the regulations were in future complied with.

The managers then called in Dr Shand and heard from him in explanation, but did not consider the explanation at all satisfactory, whereupon it was moved and universally resolved after considering the minute of the managers of 20th May and the manner in which Dr Shand had disregarded the resolution then adopted, that they had no alternative but now to discharge the very painful duty of dismissing Dr Shand from the office of resident clerk to the Infirmary, 'and he is held to be dismissed from this date'.

26 August 1844. The following letter from Dr Shand was read to the meeting of managers:

> My Lord and Gentlemen, 21 August 1844 It was with great pain that I last night received your communication discharging me from acting longer as a Resident clerk to the Infirmary. I beg to express my sincere regret at the circumstances which gave rise to this and to assure you that they arose not from any feeling of disrespect towards your honourable board nor from any intention of treating your regulations lightly, but rather from inadvertancy. I would fain hope that under all the circumstances of the case your honourable board may still find it open to reconsider a decision which may have so very injurious an effect upon the prospects of a young man like myself, just about to enter on his

profession. And allow me to add that should you be pleased to restore me to my place among the clerks, I shall take care that there shall be no room for any complaint against me hereafter for infringing the law in question.

I have the honour to be, My Lord and Gentlemen, Your most obedient humble servant,

(signed) John Shand

I beg leave to append a statement of the following facts which, although they do not excuse, may I trust serve to palliate my conduct.

Statement

Last week I was once beyond hours. On the 13th I was prevented from returning till one a.m. in consequence of visiting friends of mine who had come here from a great distance and who were spending a few days in the neighbourhood, three or four miles from town. As the evening was exceedingly wet, I was induced to remain some little time in hopes of the weather clearing.

On the 17th when I was late I previously gave notice to the Superintendent of the probability of my being out over hours. This week again, on Sunday last, I was late but reached the Infirmary before twelve. This certainly I shall take care shall not occur again.

Permit me to mention that I have acted as a Resident clerk for nearly a twelvemonth preceding this date and previous to that I was employed as a non-resident clerk and Dresser for a nearly equal period. For the manner in which I have discharged my duties I beg to refer to Mr Syme, Dr Duncan, Dr Handyside, Dr Robertson and Professor Miller whose names I give in the order I have served under them in your establishment.

James Shand

The meeting having anxiously deliberated on this important matter were unanimously of the opinion that while on the one hand the resolution of the former meeting was absolutely necessary with a view to the due observation of the rules and regulations of the Institution, it now appeared to them that, in consequence of the statement made by Dr Shand in which he acknowledged the impropriety of his conduct and pledged himself in the event of his being restored to his situation to give proper obedience to the regulations of the managers, and further, in consequence of the very favourable account which the managers have received from different quarters of the previous good conduct of Dr Shand, they are justified in reponing him against the resolution which had been adopted, and accordingly restore Dr Shand to the situation of resident clerk, and it is anxiously hoped that the future good conduct of Dr Shand and his brother clerks will prevent the recurrence of so very painful a measure on the part of the managers.

Dr Shand wrote to the managers seven days later, requesting 'a few weeks leave'. He was told he could have four weeks leave but not until one of the two clerks presently on holiday returned. After his leave he applied to have his period as resident clerk extended. This was agreed to with a reminder of his previous undertakings.

25 November 1844. Dr Handyside complained to the managers that his clerk, Dr Fleming, had published a case without reference to the conditions Dr Handyside had set for publication. Dr Fleming was heard in explanation. A letter of regret was sent to Dr Handyside.

28 January 1845. A special meeting of the board was held at the request of the House Committee. The House Committee complained that Drs Dickson and Combe, on the night of 22–3 January, had got access to the hospital at a late hour by clambering over the wall and rails and entering by a window. The managers in their deliberations noted that if the clerks were dismissed 'it would be a severe blow to their parents, who are well-known and highly respectable citizens of Edinburgh and Leith respectively. The six resident clerks were then called in, as were the two apprentices in the laboratory, and were addressed by the chairman in the presence of the managers, the treasurer-superintendent, the clerk, the matron, the chaplain and the apothecary.' Drs. Dickson and Combe were admonished for their 'extreme impropriety'.

11 November 1844. The clerks, along with other appointees to the Infirmary, had to take the 'Oath de fidèle' on appointment. Their presence in the hospital was subsequently carefully regulated. An exception to the number required to be in the building was allowed on the evening of the weekly Medical Society meeting, when it was agreed that only one clerk need be in the hospital. His name, however, was to be in a book at the porter's lodge.

10 March 1845. Too many patients were being admitted. 'The managers were very displeased to find that in some cases this was being done by placing two patients (full grown men) in the same bed.' At the same meeting, after more accounts of the late nights of the clerks, the question was asked 'Are the clerks in the habit of visiting their respective wards between 7 and 9 am?' The answer is not recorded.

31 March 1845. Dr John Struthers was reprimanded for allowing there to be eleven instead of nine patients in ward 4 (Prof. Miller), although the extras were accident cases. He was told that he must use available beds in other surgical wards before doing this, and told that he would face dismissal if the situation occurred again. He must communicate with the clerks of the other wards.

31 July 1845. Dr Fleming had written a book [*sic*] criticising the use of antimony in the medical wards of Edinburgh Royal. This was investigated by the managers who found that awareness of the dangers of antimony was 'clear to all workers'. They also found that 'Dr Fleming watched patients well as a clerk'. Only four patients had reached what Dr Fleming had called the 'fourth degree of operation' and in none was the effect designed. No further case could have been seen by Dr Fleming as there were none. Dr Fleming was now satisfied that he had erred on this issue. Reprints of his book would be 'leaving out the more objectionable sentiments which were calculated to lead to misconception on the part of the public.'

16 February 1846. The clerks again in trouble, this time because of 'unauthorised visitors to their quarters' and because 'three clerks of the Surgical Hospital had all been out at the same time on the night of 23 January'. There were no serious repercussions.

31 May 1847. A clerk, William McDougall, died of 'fever'.

19 July 1847. 'The clerks were called in and congratulated on their behaviour and work.'

1 February 1848. William Tennant Gairdner [a major star of the future] was spoken to by authority, as 'he had been out twice beyond hours in the past week'.

14 March 1848. A letter had been received by Mr Hope, the solicitor member of the Infirmary board, from a gentleman who had sent his servant in to hospital on Tuesday 7 March. He claimed she was not seen in the ward until the Thursday. The ward, the Servants' ward, was temporarily in the charge of Dr Andrew, covering for a colleague. An explanation was sought by Mr Hope.

Dr Andrew said he saw the woman in the waiting room, diagnosed mild erysipelas of the face and did not think she required any treatment 'other than a mild laxative'. He saw her again on the Thursday, being away from the hospital on the Wednesday. As was normal practice, he assumed that his clerk, Dr Haldane, would cover his duties as well as his own. In reply to a further charge that another woman, Agnes Craik, died in that ward on that Wednesday, Dr Andrew said that when he saw her on the Tuesday 'she was in a state of severe and exhausting hectic [*sic*] which I was satisfied would soon prove fatal'.

Dr Haldane explained that he had been ill on these days and left his bed only to attend the most ill patients in the other wards under his care. The nurse in the servants' ward did not tell him of the new admission or he would have seen her too.

Mr Hope then moved that Dr Haldane be dismissed but there was no seconder. Mr Baillie, the Faculty of Advocates representative on the board, moved that Dr Haldane be reprimanded. This was agreed to, Hope dissenting. Dr Haldane was asked to appear before the managers at their next meeting. At that meeting he was reprimanded in front of the other clerks, who had been required to be present. Shortly after, Haldane was granted two weeks sick leave.

A protest letter from Dr Andrew's colleagues was dismissed on the basis that the ultimate responsibility for daily ward visiting lies with the senior doctor of the ward. He had been told by the board that 'they regretted very much that he did not arrange cover . . . ' Hope was not pleased with these findings. He put it on record that 'he hoped that, with reference to the ward complained of, Dr Paterson would return as soon as possible to its care'.

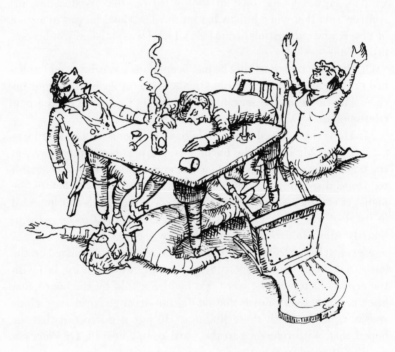

❧ 8 ❧

Edinburgh and the Beginning of Anaesthesia

The drowsy syrups of the world shall
medicine thee to that sweet sleep.

SHAKESPEARE, *Othello*

One or two pennyworth of gin might have meant a good evening out in an Edinburgh hostelry in 1840. Administered instead in the operating theatre of the city's Royal Infirmary, and accompanied by a blindfold and a leather gag, it seems barely enough to ensure the cooperation of a man about to have his leg amputated. This was, however, the anaesthesia of the early 1840s, sometimes accompanied by laudanum, a non-standardised opiate inadequate for the purpose. Some had even tried hypnosis. The expression 'to bite the bullet' dates from these times, a soldier being handed a lead bullet on which to bite when undergoing surgery in the field. Later in the decade ether and chloroform came into use.

The SS *Arcadia* arrived in Liverpool from the USA in early December 1846. In Boston her surgeon Dr Fraser had witnessed the removal of a vascular tumour under ether anaesthesia. Much impressed, he left the ship immediately she docked and brought the news to his home town of Dumfries in the south of Scotland. There, on 19 December 1846, Britain's first surgery under ether took place. Two days later in London, Dr Liston, who trained in Edinburgh, performed an amputation on Robert Churchill, a butler, also under ether. Liston, having finished the operation, said 'This Yankee dodge, gentlemen, beats mesmerism hollow!'

Liston's news spread quickly. He wrote to his friend Professor Miller, one of the two professors of surgery in Edinburgh. On 23 December Miller read the letter to his students and informed his Queen Street neighbour, the obstetrician James Young Simpson. Before the year ended, Simpson was in London talking to Liston.

During 1847 Simpson used ether in all his cases in Edinburgh's lying-in hospital in the Canongate. 'Sleep is sweet to the labouring man', said Bunyan in *Pilgrim's Progress* to which Simpson, a humane obstetrician, would probably have added ' . . . and labouring woman'. The surgical wards in the Royal Infirmary began to use ether in the same year but worries about its safety arose. 'The arterial blood becomes black and a few deaths have occurred' a London surgeon wrote to Simpson. A safer substance was required. Simpson found it.

The story of Simpson's introduction of chloroform as an anaesthetic is well known. Some of the preliminary testing was carried out at his home at 52 Queen Street, Edinburgh in October 1847. Drs Simpson, George Keith and Matthews Duncan had been trying out various substances they thought might be useful by sniffing them and noting their effects. One evening they tried chloroform, supplied by the manufacturing chemists Duncan and Flockhart. Professor Miller heard of that evening soon afterwards and reported that 'hilarity was followed by sleep'. 'By 3 am,' he goes on, 'guests were very impressed. A gallant lady, Miss Agnes Petrie the family niece, tried it that evening having come down from bed on hearing the extraordinary sounds from the dining room. She was somewhat large and fat but the chloroform apparently had the marvellous effect of letting her slip out of her big body. With an ethereal look on her podgy face she folded her hands on her chest and slid to the floor crying out in ecstasy "I'm an angel, oh, an angel!" '

Chloroform was first used on 8 November 1847 in Edinburgh. Simpson gave it to a doctor's wife, Jane Carstairs, who in her last pregnancy had undergone a traumatic embryulcia. This time the delivery was normal and the baby was taken into the next room before the patient awoke. On wakening, the mother said she was afraid the sleep had stopped her pains. She had to be convinced that the delivery was over and that the baby was indeed hers.

Professor Miller was especially keen to try it on his surgical patients. Miller, an Angus man and a son of the manse, was a pupil of Liston. He was said to be handsome, eloquent and sensitive, given to sweating before operating because of the patient's pain and thus known to his students as 'the surgeon who hated to operate'. He was on the lookout for a suitable case, and a man with a strangulated hernia arrived. But Simpson could not be found, the operation went ahead with no anaesthetic and the patient died. Simpson said later that if this patient had had chloroform 'its whole career would have been arrested'.

On 10 November 1847 Miller got his chance. The gallery in theatre was full as word got round that chloroform was to be used that day. A six year old boy had 'the sequestrum of nearly the whole radius' removed under the drug. Miller's notes conclude 'Not the slightest evidence of the suffering of pain was given. He slept soundly and was carried to the ward in that state. Half an hour later he was awake with a clear merry eye and a placid expression of countenance, wholly unlike what is found to obtain after ordinary etherisation. On being questioned he said he had felt no pain and felt none now. On being shown his wounded arm he looked surprised'.

Simpson's pamphlet on chloroform was published five days after this operation. It bore the words of Bacon 'I esteem it the office of a physician, not only to restore health but to mitigate pain and dolor'. The pamphlet was dedicated to the chemist Professor Dumas, Dean of the Faculty of Science in Paris, who had been at the operation. Dumas was the first to work out the chemical composition of the new anaesthetic. Four thousand copies of Simpson's pamphlet were sold in a few days and many thousands later.

By 1850 chloroform had been used in almost one hundred thousand patients in Edinburgh alone. In 1853 it was used in the delivery of one of Queen Victoria's children. Simpson claimed that he had no deaths from chloroform till 1870 but was said to have suppressed some. One such was Mrs H. who died while having teeth extracted. Simpson put her death down to excitement, but it was believed by others to be due to chloroform. Lister recorded that Professor Syme, for many years Scotland's leading surgeon, had performed five thousand operations under chloroform by 1861, with no deaths due to the anaesthetic.

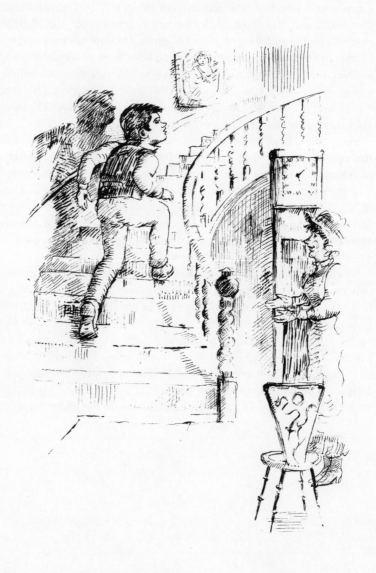

❧ 9 ❧

One of the Physicians

'Physicians of the utmost fame
Were called at once; but when they came
They answered, as they took their fees,
"There is no cure for this disease."'
HILAIRE BELLOC, 'Henry King' (1907)

'Run upstairs, Robert, and tell your father that Nelson's dead. Tell him we've just had a great victory off Cape Trafalgar!' The year was 1805 and Christison senior was temporarily ill in the family's Forfarshire home.

The young Robert Christison, who in his autobiography reported this as his earliest memory, was to become a well-known and conscientious physician in Edinburgh Royal Infirmary. His career was a long one. He earned the title of 'physician of two generations' partly because of his many years in the Infirmary and partly because of the objectivity which characterised his progress throughout. He is said to have willingly accepted changing ideas in medicine, particularly with regard to therapeutics.

By a coincidence it fell to Christison to examine one of the bodies the infamous Burke had provided for Dr Knox the anatomist. The police had intercepted the body in transit and Christison confirmed that death was due to strangulation, not smothering as claimed. On his appointment as professor of materia medica and medical jurisprudence he became the Crown's usual expert witness in poisoning cases. This included his appearance in the well-known Madeleine Smith murder case in 1857. He died in 1882 three years after the opening of the new Royal Infirmary in the Meadows. He had been one of the speakers at the ceremony. In the blunt style of the time William Tennant Gairdner, in an obituary, felt able to include the sentence 'Christison was a reserved man, totally committed to his patients, but also of an *hauteur* which was perhaps not quite favourable to a rapid or extreme success in private practice'.

A kindlier story is told by a Dr John Ross, who thought it illustrative of his friend's 'affectionate thoughtfulness'. 'Christison's wife, a woman of great beauty and *better* [*sic*], was in her last illness. She was going to the country for a month and her husband heard her give orders that a piece of worsted work, which she had finished, should be grounded and made up as an ottoman, and ready in the drawing room on her return. A few days before her return he asked if it was completed: it had been totally forgotten. He said nothing but, getting possession of the piece, he sat up for two or three nights and grounded it with his own hands, had it made up, and sat his wife down on it as she had wished.'

THE BRITISH PHARMACOPOEIA

While Christison's whole working life was spent in Edinburgh, his contribution to British medicine was recognised by the award of a knighthood. He helped in the preparation of the last edition of the Edinburgh Pharmacopoeia in 1841 and contributed an account of its history to the *Edinburgh Medical Journal* [1842, p. 501]. He was appointed chairman of the Medical Council committee that had been instructed to draw up a new pharmacopoeia for use in the whole of Britain. This amalgamation of the pharmacopoeias of England, Scotland and Ireland was to be the first edition of the *British Pharmacopoeia*. An Act of Parliament stated it was to be substituted for the several regional pharmacopoeias then in use. This was a good move allowing standardisation of names. Its usefulness can be seen in some of the prescriptions referred to in this book.

Christison had the reputation of being adaptable to changes in medical thinking. On at least two important matters during the 1840s, he made others aware of serious therapeutic dangers. He worried about the current treatment of syphilis. The Infirmary had a 'salivation ward' for patients with this disease (see chapter on 'The Layout of the Infirmary'). Christison's experience there led him to become anxious about the toxic effects of mercury, the most commonly used substance in the treatment of syphilis. He pointed out the dangers of 'mercurio-syphilis and mercuric cachexia'. Again, somewhat later, he made a valuable contribution when he raised doubts about the extensive use of blood-letting in its several forms, as a non-specific therapeutic technique.

HIS VIEWS ON SCURVY AND 'FEVER'

On scurvy he was wrong. Surprisingly the advice he gave in the mid-1840s, when called in to advise on an outbreak of the disease in Perth Prison, made no reference to the provision of fruit and vegetables. Details of this and his comments on a different outbreak are discussed in the next chapter.

On the aetiology of the fever or fevers which caused the Scottish epidemics of the nineteenth century his views were again controversial. It is true, however, that the subject confused many physicians over many years. Writing on his older colleague's death in 1882, William Tennant Gairdner described Christison's approach to the matter as, 'for once *not* that of the physician of two generations'.

The clinical management of the thousands of fever victims was not affected by the diagnostic uncertainty. Christison and his colleagues had, indeed, no specific treatment to offer. The need was essentially for good nursing care. All Infirmary staff spent long hours in the wards but, unlike most of his fellows, Christison also held a University chair. This meant he had to find time for teaching, and administration as well as for his work in the wards. It was an exhausting burden. In a lighter mood Christison told a story in his autobiography which showed that doctors and nurses are no more immune to illness than anyone else:

> During the 1842 epidemic I visited an ailing friend, Dr Hughes Bennett. I told him he was suffering from my old friend, the recurring form of synocha, which I recognised from 1817 and 1827. I warned Bennett that he would suffer a recurrence before the fourteenth day. Bennett smiled and said 'There isn't time to be lost by it then! It is now 3 p.m. and the fourteenth day will end in five hours. For I was taken ill quite abruptly at eight in the evening this day fortnight!' I went straight home to Randolph Crescent, about one mile. Next day I learned that I could scarcely have reached my door before Bennett was attacked with violent rigors and then by crisis and profuse sweating. The students, who have a trick of eliciting a joke out of any remarkable incident, insisted I had practised on his self-suggestion, on the influence of which, in causing and curing disease, Dr Bennett had several times been learnedly discoursing at this period!

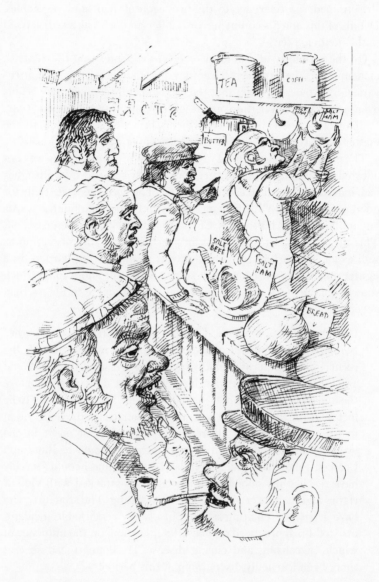

❧ 10 ❧

'A Disease almost Unknown in these Parts . . . '

My living in Yorkshire was so far out of the way that it
was actually twelve miles from a lemon!
REV. SYDNEY SMITH, *Lady Holland's Memoir*

Already under great pressure to find accommodation for fever
patients, and with an outbreak of dysentery in both medical and
surgical wards, the Infirmary authorities in the crisis year of 1847
had to cope with another rush of admissions. Two hundred and forty
nine extra people were admitted between 1 January and 29 April,
suffering from a disease described by a board member as 'almost
unknown in this part of the world'.

The disease was scurvy, the cause dietary deficiency of ascorbic
acid (vitamin C). While scurvy was not, in fact, at all unknown in
Edinburgh, the number of patients was extraordinary. Most of them
came from the railway construction camps on the moors around
Edinburgh. (The Infirmary's other difficulties with the rapid de-
velop- ment of the railways are described in a later chapter.) These
camps were isolated and a large number of the workmen were Irish
with no permanent Scottish home. Many men, therefore, lived for
long periods in these remote places, consuming only the food the
railway companies provided for them. This was available only at the
companies' on-site stores. What it consisted of is recorded in the
case records which follow. It was lacking in variety. The need for
fresh fruit and vegetables was either not understood or they were too
expensive or difficult to bring in. Of more importance there was an
absence of potatoes due to continuing crop failures. In 1845 half the
potato crop in Ireland was lost. In 1846 almost all the Irish and
British crop was lost. As potatoes would normally provide the
vitamin C in a labourer's diet in an isolated situation such as this,
scurvy was almost inevitable. In the city potatoes were also short,
which probably explains the weaver Brand's illness. The total

number of admissions was high this being even more remarkable when it is realised that normal body stores of the vitamin will last for up to six months after deprivation begins! Labourers Dermot McCulloch, Bernard Cairns and George Doyle gave typical histories.

The Royal Navy had in 1795 eradicated scurvy from its ships (see below). The information about how this was achieved appears to have been very slow to spread beyond that service. Harold Strang, for example, was a merchant seaman from Leith who was admitted to the Infirmary – for other reasons – in 1848, i.e. fifty-three years later. He had been employed in the whale fishery for six years and was now a deckhand on the Edinburgh–Burntisland ferry. 'Last summer,' his notes record, 'scurvy broke out among the whaling crew at Greenland . . .'

The board, as usual, coped successfully with the need for more accommodation. The minutes of 19 April 1847 note that: 'The large wooden shed is to be opened for the accommodation of these labourers with scurvy.' The board wished the three railway boards to pay the costs of their employees' admissions. 'To this date' the minutes say, 'from 1 March, there have been 173 cases from the North British branch to Hawick, 45 from the Caledonian and 31 from the Edinburgh and Northern.' A letter to the railway boards included the passage: 'In the opinion of the medical men the diseases with which the men are afflicted have been brought on by the character of the diet on which they have subsisted.' It was suggested that the only treatment needed was that the men 'be fed in a different manner, which could equally well be done in the country'. There was no specific advice on what food should be provided.

There are inconsistencies in Edinburgh's management of scurvy at this time which are surprising in the city in which Lind, in 1753, published the original ' Treatise on the Scurvy'.

DERMOT MCCULLOCH, aged 29
Crighton Moss (ex-Donegal). Railway labourer.
21 March 1847. Admitted to Edinburgh Royal Infirmary. His mental faculties seem very obtuse and considerable difficulty is experienced in drawing from him his history. For many years he has been employed as a railway labourer in various places. Last

summer he was working at Middleton Muir. Subsequently on the North British line at Alnwick. More recently he was about three months at St Boswell's Green and for the last two to three weeks he has been again on the Hawick line at Middleton Muir. Has always got his provisions, consisting of bread, tea, salt ham and beef from contractor's stores. Sometimes good, sometimes bad. On the whole does not complain much of the quality of his food. Sometimes took salt meat every day in the week. Sometimes none in a week. No idea how long a pound of ham lasted. A loaf of bread generally served four or five times.

Six or seven weeks ago complained of pain and swelling in the ham of the left leg. This has increased. Gums tender, swollen and bleeding. The whole left leg and ankle swollen, painful blue in colour and hard. Many purple spots.

℞ To have full diet. *Int: balneum tepidum vespere.*[1]

19 April 1847. To have a flannel bandage applied

10 May 1847. Dismissed cured.[2]   I. Robertson

BERNARD CAIRNS, aged 20

Middleton Muir. Labourer.

15 March 1847. Admitted to Medical Ward. Has been working at Middleton Muir on the Hawick line of railway for upwards of a year. Has always been supplied with provisions at a store for behoof of the labourers. For many months the provisions were of a very bad quality so much so that at last the workers in a body resisted taking them. A new store was established since when the articles have been, on the whole, better though frequently anything but excellent. The diet has consisted exclusively of bread, salt, butter, tea, sometimes coffee with sugar but without milk. Salt ham and salt beef generally not more than twice a week. The bread was often very bad. A loaf lasted three, sometimes four times. He cannot tell how long a pound of ham lasted. He has been off work for five weeks having been obliged to stop by frost which interrupted the work, and prevented from resuming it from pain

---

[1] 'To have a tepid bath every second evening.'

[2] Note duration of admission.

in the lower parts of both legs, especially the right. Some time after this his gums became much swelled and very tender, of a purple color and bleeding on being touched. He has been in Edinburgh about a week and has taken chiefly porridge and milk with some eggs since that time.

On examination his gums are much less swelled than formerly and the dark colour has nearly gone, the improvement having taken place in the last day or two. They are still however a little tender and easily made to bleed. Both legs are somewhat swelled and hard. Several small dark spots may be seen round the roots of the hairs in the right ham. He complains of much pain and stiffness in the legs.

℞ *Sumat Tinct: Opii.*[1]

20 March 1847. Int: balneum tepidum alterno qq nocte.[2]

29 March 1847. A flannel bandage for each leg.

12 April 1847. Dismissed cured.

GEORGE DOYLE, aged 21

Middleton Muir (ex-Donegal). Railway navvy.

10 April 1847. Admitted to hospital. Since July has worked at Middleton Muir . . . [He describes his diet in the same words as Cairns. His signs are the same]

℞ To have full diet.

15 May 1847. ℞ *Succi Limonum* 3 oz. *Sacchar.* 1½ oz. *Aq.* 2 oz. *Solve et sumat pro potu in aqua in dies.*[3]

22 May 1847. Dismissed cured.[4]   I. Robertson

[1] 'To have Tincture of Opium'.

[2] 'A tepid bath to be taken on alternate nights.'

[3] This is a mixture of lemon juice, sugar and water. The instruction means 'Dissolve and take as a drink in water daily.'

[4] He was prescribed a full diet on admission but it was five weeks before lemon juice was added. The diet alone would have cured him, more slowly, and was doing so as he was dismissed 'cured' only one week after the lemon juice was added. The delay in prescribing the specific cure is odd.

JAMES BRAND, aged 34

Cowgate, ex-Ireland (Drogheda). A weaver.

7 April 1847. Admitted with a two week history of sore gums. Living principally on bread and tea with fresh meat two or three times a week. Sometimes porridge but never had milk to it. Took about 1 lb. of bread at a meal. Leg pains. Bruises. Gums spongy. ℞ *Calcis chlorinat.* 2 drachms. *Aqua* 10 oz. *M. Sol: Col: Lav: os. internum saepe.*[1]

13 April 1847. Better.

8 May 1847. Liq: Alumis 2 drachms. *Aqua* 8 ounces *Fiat gargarisma.*[2] *Habeat balneum tepidum vespere.*[3]

25 May 1847. Dismissed cured.   I. Robertson

[1] Although 'calcis chlorinat:' means 'chlorinated lime' this has nothing to do with the citrus version of 'lime'! Calcis chlorinat: possesses bleaching and disinfecting properties and was here used as a mouthwash or collutorium for his spongy gums; 'M. Sol: Col:' means 'provide a collutorium solution' i.e. a mouthwash solution. The instruction is 'wash the inside of the mouth frequently'. As his spongy gums were due to scurvy he would have been better off with the citrus kind of lime. This is the fruit that led to Royal Navy sailors being called 'Limeys'.

[2] 'Make a gargle.' Alum, the sulphate of alumina and potash, was astringent and had many uses. As a gargle, Beasley says it was used for 'relaxed sore throat, excessive salivation etc.'.

[3] 'To have a tepid bath in the evening'.

TREATMENT OF SCURVY—A SURPRISING STORY

It seems very odd that, although Lind in 1753 and Cook in 1755 realised that scurvy could be treated with oranges, limes and lemons, this prophylactic and effective treatment took so long to be permanently accepted. In 1795 the Admiralty made the issue of three-quarters of an ounce of lemon juice per man per day compulsory in the Royal Navy. The disease was thus eradicated on long voyages. No fewer than 1.6 million gallons of lemon juice were issued between 1795 and 1814 (Lloyd and Coulter, *Medicine in the Navy, 1200-1900,* Vol. 3, 1714–1815, Edinburgh, Livingstone).

Perth Prison suffered an outbreak of scurvy in 1845–6. Dr Robert Christison, the physician, was asked to advise. His advice, given half a century after the Admiralty's successful order, and nearly one hundred years after Lind's first paper, surprisingly made no mention of fruit or vegetables.

Christison wrote again on scurvy during the railway construction camp outbreak in 1847. In the *Monthly Journal of Medical Science*, vii, 1847, p. 873, and vii, 1848, p.1, he suggested that the scurvy epidemic was due to 'deficiency in the nitrogenous principles in the food' the diet being too purely farinaceous, saccharo-farinaceous or saccharo-farinaceous and fatty; that this tendency cannot be counteracted by even a superabundance of the vegetable nitrogenous principle, gluten; but that it may be effectively counteracted by milk and probably also by the nitrogenised articles of food from the animal world'. But he added that others got scurvy when 'they had too much animal nutriment'. It is difficult to escape the conclusion that he was confused. A Dr Anderson from Glasgow, a Dr Curran from Dublin and a Dr Lonsdale from 'NW England' all published replies to Christison rebutting his remarks. Anderson, for example, was sure scurvy was 'not due to lack of nitrogenous compounds because it responded so well to lemon juice'. It is again odd that, at the very time that Christison's paper appeared, lemon juice was being given to George Doyle and at least some other scurvy patients in the medical wards of Edinburgh Royal Infirmary.

A Footnote

Athough nothing to do with the Infirmary and the 1840s, it is interesting to find that several men on Captain Scott's 1901 South Pole expedition suffered from scurvy. Lime and lemon juice were on board but only some men took them regularly. Scott was a regular naval officer and must have been aware of how the Admiralty had eradicated the disease. In *The Voyage of the Discovery* he describes his own spongy, bleeding gums and painful swollen legs.

Scott's problem was that he still believed that scurvy was due to something in the diet, not to something missing from it. And this was on a ship where those men who had been taking lime juice regularly were free from the disease. Scott wrote: 'It is easy to see that many cures might have been attributed to the virtues of supposed antidotes, which were really due to discontinuance of the article of food that caused the disease.' His suspicions centred on tinned meat and on bacon. He ordered perfectly good stocks of the former to be destroyed.

Unwittingly he eventually did the right thing. He tells in *The Voyage of the* Discovery how he 'took the cook in hand and insisted that the men ate seal meat. The issue of bottled fruits is to be increased and mustard and cress grown for sufferers. Lime juice is to be placed on mess tables at dinner'. One of *Discovery's* doctors, Wilson, later wrote in the *British Medical Journal*: 'We at no time forced lemon juice, increasing instead the ration of jam and bottled fruit, but lime juice was freely taken by many of the men who liked it. In some it disagreed and in my own case marked symptoms were got rid off with no lime juice'. He attributed everyone's recovery 'primarily to eating fresh seal meat twice daily, six days a week'. Scott saw his men recover and, in October 1902 wrote, 'Somewhere in this, but not wholly revealed, lies the root of our scurvy trouble; one would fain be able to trace it more clearly'.

Unsurprisingly he did not know that seals, in contrast to man, can make their own ascorbic acid (man's vitamin C). It is found, however, only in their livers. So, while seal meat does not contain the substance, seal liver does. Scott said most of *Discovery's* men found seal meat unappetising, especially when eaten twelve times a week. It is as well, therefore, that they did not know it was of no benefit to their scurvy unless they ate the liver. They were cured by the combination of the lime juice on the table at dinner, the bottled fruit, depending on its type, and seal liver. How much better it would have been if they had all stuck from the beginning to the Royal Navy's well-established practice of a daily issue of lime juice.

UNUSUAL CASES FROM THE JOURNALS: II

PATRICK CRAIGIE, aged 51
Fishmarket Close. A labourer.
18 June 1844. Admitted to surgical wards of Professor Syme.

Two years ago, while lifting a heavy weight, he felt something give way and observed at the same time a tumour on his left groin. He never observed any change in the size of this tumour, nor did he experience any inconvenience from it till about one month ago. It then became somewhat harder, accompanied by costiveness of the bowels and pain, more particularly of the part but extending over the whole abdomen with a feeling of hardness and distension.

On examination there is an irreducible hernia about the size of a hen's egg.

22 June 1844. By frequent attempts to reduce the hernia above mentioned, the size has diminished to about that of a walnut, consisting entirely of omentum. The application of a truss effectively prevents the coming down of the gut. Dismissed relieved.   K. K.

OTTO LAHR, aged 55
From Germany. A travelling spectacle salesman.
7 May 1841. Admitted to Professor Syme's wards.

Has much pain in the region of the anus. Two years ago first felt pain in this part on going to stool and was unable to sit on a chair with comfort. Constipation was the original cause of his symptoms, he supposes, and they have gone on becoming worse and worse ever since.

External and internal haemorrhoids are present. The former are larger. The latter appear at the centre of the protrusion and are of a bright red colour and of small cutens.[2]

15 June 1841. Dismissed cured after operation.   R. M.

---

[1] Operative treatment of hernia was not yet being performed.

[2] 'Cutens' means 'skin covering'.

STEVEN MCLEAN, aged 39
Crossford, Dunfermline. A weaver.
8 August 1844. Admitted to surgical wards of Professor Syme.

For the last eight or nine years a small firm moveable tumour has existed in the left hip, situated nearly over the tuberosity of the ischium. During the last eight months it has rapidly increased in size. It is now the size of a small apple.

9 August 1844. The tumour was today dissected out and found to consist of a cyst containing atheromatous matter.

19 August 1844. Dismissed cured.   M.C.

BIDDY REID, aged 13
House of Refuge. Father dead.
29 April 1841. Admitted to Professor Syme's care on account of the effects of frostbite. In the month of December last she was much exposed to extreme cold and damp. The effect was pain, swelling and red discolouration of the toes and metatarsi of her left foot, also of three of her right toes. Since that period, the parts of the left foot have separated and now an ulcerated stump alone exists in this situation. The third right toe is also much ulcerated and the whole parts are the seat of great pain.
Poultice to be applied.

2 May 1841. The sores are now freed from the unhealthy looking matter which covered them. Poultices discontinued and sulphate of zinc lotion to be applied.[2]

13 June 1841. The parts have now entirely cicatrised and formed an ample covering for the bones.

29 June 1841. Dismissed cured.   R. McKenzie

---

[1] This might have been an ischial tuberosity bursitis, caused by prolonged sitting on a hard surface. In even earlier times, the weavers' habit of sitting cross-legged at work had led to this condition becoming known as 'weaver's bottom.'

[2] Sulphate of zinc lotion was 'one of the best astringents known'. (Beasley)

MARGARET MACLEOD, aged 22
Isle of Skye
8 July 1841. Admitted to Professor Syme's care. She is from the Isle of Skye and cannot speak English.[1]

Two years ago she cut the inner part of the tendon of the heel with a scythe. The wound remained open and at the end of twelve months numerous small pieces of bone of the size of pinheads were discharged. The sore has since remained open but has not caused much pain or inconvenience.

On examination there exists a small callous [*sic*] ulcer over the inner side of the os calcis. On introducing a probe, small loose pieces of bone are felt.

12 July 1841. An incision was made over the part of the bone where the loose pieces of bone are felt and several small portions (not much larger than barley corns) were taken out.

26 July 1841. Dismissed cured.

Entry in ward journal reads – caries of *os calcis.* Diseased bone removed by operation.

MARIA BLAIR, aged 20
A servant, from Aberdeen
24 August 1848. Admitted to Ward 11. States that she arrived in Leith from the north on Sunday 20th. Was seasick during the voyage. Before leaving home had been attending her sister's husband who died a fortnight ago of 'the fever'. On Tuesday last (two days ago) had a severe headache which had been slight the day before; felt cold but had no distinct rigor. Has been getting worse since.

On examination the face is of a bright scarlet colour as is also the lower part of the neck. On both arms there are large patches of a bright scarlet colour, irregular in shape and from two to four inches square. On the chest and abdomen there are numerous small bright red spots, the largest crowned by a small, slightly raised vesicle, about the size of a small pin's head. Skin very hot;

[1] People who could speak only Gaelic were to be found in the Hebrides until at least the mid-1960s. Even at the end of the 1990s there are many who regard English as very much their second language.

pungent in some parts. Tongue white with a thick fur through which, towards the point, bright red papillae project. Throat red and tender. Pulse full, about 100. She complains of severe frontal headache; has great thirst and loss of appetite.

Applic: hirudines 8 temporibus.

℞ *Matur pulv: effervescens et hab statim pulv: jalap comp:* ½ drachm.[1]

25 August 1848. Headache somewhat better. Pain in throat.

Urine of a brownish red colour. SG 1022. Rendered muddy by heat; cleared slightly at first by nitric acid which causes coagulation in form of diffused granular particles. On standing, the urine deposited a dense nut-brown sediment occupying about a quarter of the vessel. This consisted (under the microscope) of a brownish granular matter. No organic substance perceptible.

29 August 1848. ℞ *Sol: ammoniae acetatis* 2 oz. *Sp: etheris nitrici* 3 drachms. *Aqua* 6 oz. *Sumat* ½ oz. *tertia quaque.*[2]

2 Oct [*sic*] Having gone on favourably she was dismissed cured.

J. S.

The index of the ward journal gives the diagnosis in this case as scarletina.

---

[1] The cathartic, Jalapa, a Mexican root, had many uses but a Dr Hamilton is quoted by Beasley as using it specifically in Scarletina, in combination with Aquae Canellae. The latter was derived from a West Indian tree. The instruction here is 'make an effervescent powder of Compound Powder of Jalap and have half a drachm at once.'

[2] Acetate of ammonia and the ether preparation are both stated by Beasley to be used as diaphoretics and diuretics.

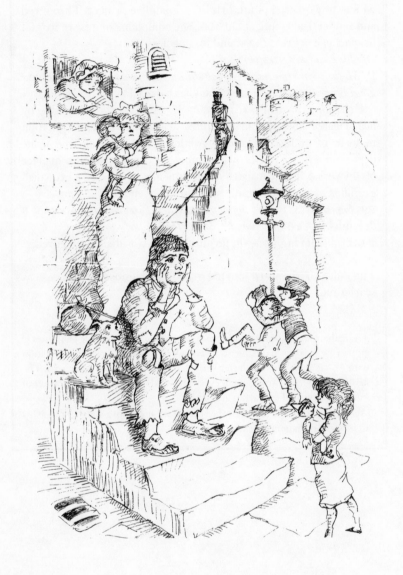

Poverty in Edinburgh

The awful phantom of the hungry poor.
HARRIET B. SPOFFER, *A Winter's Night*

Andrew McPhail was a fifty-five year old sheep shearer. He lived in a primitive barn near the shore, outside Edinburgh. 'Lumbago had stopped him working, and for six months he has been living on shellfish which were boiled before eating. Seldom or never got a dish of porridge.' On admission to the Infirmary he showed signs of malnutrition and was ordered 'to have a full diet including porridge with milk'.

Charles Robertson, aged forty-nine, was admitted from the House of Refuge. A labourer to trade he was originally from Newcastle. He had come north to seek employment four weeks before admission. However 'since his arrival he has been out of work and in extreme destitution, sleeping nightly at the House of Refuge and living upon very poor diet'. He also was prescribed a full diet.

Both these men were in hospital, not with a specific illness, but as members of the hungry poor. They were dealt with compassionately, being kept in hospital long enough for a proper diet to produce benefit. The cost of this prolonged support was borne by the same people who voluntarily provided all the funds required to run the Infirmary, namely the local population.

There remained some, however, to whom the poor seemed a curiosity if not almost a different species. This attitude was reflected in one anonymous verse:

> Whene'er I walk this beauteous earth
> How many poor I see
> But as I never speaks to them
> They never speaks to me.

A very odd little book called *Low Life in Victorian Edinburgh* written by a 'Medical Gentleman' exemplified this approach. The publisher's introduction to the 1980 reprint suggests that, while the book draws attention to the misery of many, there is also a feeling that the author and his friend in exploring the poor areas, did so 'as if eagerly seeking a source of nineteenth century titillation'.

The book describes the scene around the Castle and in the narrow wynds, closes and vennels of the High Street and the Canongate. 'Saturday night in the High Street and Canongate of Edinburgh', it says, 'presents one of the most revolting sights ever witnessed. The filth, degradation and hopeless misery is awful and could not be exceeded: indeed it may be gravely questioned if in any city, in one night of the week, destitution, prostitution and crime, ever held such a review as they hold in the High Street of the Modern Athens'.

The writer and his companion walked through Blackfriars' Wynd during one of the fever epidemics. 'We came to a building more ruinous and dilapidated than any we had yet entered. The very stone steps of the stairs were worn away so much as considerably to impede our progress in the ascent, and descending was positively not safe. Most of the apartments nearest the staircase were untenanted, at least during the day. At night, we were told that many a houseless wanderer sought refuge from the rain and snow in their dark and dirty corners. In one house lived eighteen individuals at least. In the flat above, the effects of filth and no ventilation, sufficiently appeared, for there fever revelled. Of a family of five only the father had escaped, the mother being dangerously ill at the time of our visit. For a worse case we take the liberty of quoting from the Scotsman newspaper of so old a date as 28 November 1843. "The most distressing case, however, occurred on Tuesday. A young girl, about eleven years of age, was found in a virulent stage of the fever, lying in a small room on a common stair at the head of the Canongate, without a friend or attendant to look after her. She had previously subsisted by begging but being attacked by the prevalent disease, she crept into this empty closet where the inhabitants of the stair (with the filthy habits which have long been the reproach of Scotland) had been accustomed to empty their ashes etc. instead of carrying then down to the street. In this place she had remained from the Friday till the Tuesday, without attendance of any kind and without any supply of food or water, some of the neighbours actually throwing their ashes upon her person. She was finally noticed by some of the more humane neighbours who gave information to the police; and Dr Tait being sent for, had her removed to the Infirmary where she now remains'.

CARING FOR THE POOR

Help for the poor was, however, increasing. It consisted of two elements, the material and the financial. The town council organised most of the former, as the following extracts from Anderson's *History of Edinburgh* show.

At a public meeting in March 1840 the council sought 'to improve the conditions of the poor' and this initiative resulted in the first Poor Law Act for Scotland. Another meeting led to the opening of the 'night asylum for the houseless poor' in Old Fishmarket Close. This provided porridge at night, a bed and breakfast. People could thus sleep 'off streets and stairs'. Accommodation was for one night only although this was sometimes extended. While the Infirmary's charter defined its commitment to help 'the sick and hurt poor of Edinburgh', help for less serious ailments could be obtained from dispensaries in the city. These were usually run by medical students.

Work on the construction of the Queen's Drive around Arthur's Seat was made available for the unemployed. St John's Church in Victoria Terrace was opened for the poor. This had free seats, other churches in Edinburgh having high seat rents. Concerts were given with the entry price kept low, the aim being 'to elevate the tastes and habits of the trades classes above the resorting to public houses and gin palaces'.

The West Port, which in Stewart times had been the main entrance to the city from the north, had become the 'poorest and most dissi-pated district of Edinburgh'. The remarkable and influential Rev. Professor Chalmers of Edinburgh is said to have changed 'a dissolute area of whisky shops and publicans to an area of coffee houses and nice and clean lodging houses . . . ' The council now decided to tackle the rest of the housing problem more forcefully. Anderson says 'From the crowded and otherwise objectionable position of the houses in the Old Town of Edinburgh, light and air are to a great extent excluded. From the inadequate supply of water and the total absence of sewers in this locality, filth is accumulated in and around the dwellings of the working class and the poor, which, added to the density of the population, occasions much sickness, mortality and pauperism and that degradation of character which is usually attended by reckless disregard of the decencies of life.' It was resolved 'that a state of things so full of reproach to an enlightened and Christian people should be amended, and the means afforded to the working classes of Edinburgh of obtaining domestic accommodation suitable in comfort.'

By 1849 the Association for Improving the Lodging Houses of the Working Classes had three model lodging houses in successful operation, one in the West Port, one in the Cowgate and one in Merchant Street. During the past year 'upwards of 40,000 individuals had been accommodated with beds in these houses, with a security for their persons and property which they could not have had in the old lodging houses, and, though these buildings were in the very centre of disease in the city, not a single case of cholera had occurred'. This was real progress.

FINANCIAL PROVISION FOR THE POOR

The system of providing financial help to Scotland's poor changed with the passing of the Poor Law (Scotland) Act of 1845. Before the Act, responsibility for poor relief lay with the kirk sessions of individual parishes, the money coming from the voluntary contributions of their members. This system seems to have worked fairly well but in 1843 there was a crisis. This was because of the Disruption. Many people had become dissatisfied with practices, such as patronage, that were now seen as too common in the Established Church. Large numbers left to form the Free Church. There were thus many new congregations, which had to find money for new buildings and for the salaries of their ministers. While some wealthy donors helped it was inevitable that overall support for charitable causes was reduced. In particular voluntary donations to the old Kirk dropped sharply as its membership fell away. This new and serious difficulty in raising money for the poor led to that responsibility passing from the Church to the State. Parochial Boards were set up which, although they were still made up of local people, were now responsible to a new State body, the Board of Supervision. Poorhouses opened and Inspectors of the Poor were appointed. Some believed that a compulsory local tax should be introduced to support these innovations. Others opposed this on the grounds that there were still ethical reasons to expect communities to provide money voluntarily.

One decision of the Royal Infirmary's board showed how it cared for its most needy patients. Lord Medwyn, a judge, chaired the board meeting on 20 October 1845. He drew his fellow members' attention to a clause in the new Poor Law Act which made it imperative for the Inspector of the Poor to afford a poor person more ready access to relief. Medwyn thought this would imply that, on discharge from the Infirmary, someone entitled to relief would also be entitled to interim maintenance from the city's poor fund. The board therefore agreed that, to avoid delay in providing support outside hospital, 'it would be a proper and crowning act of charity to poor persons if, on their discharge from hospital, the treasurer superintendent were to send a memorandum along with them to the inspector of the poor of the city stating that they are indeed entitled to relief'.

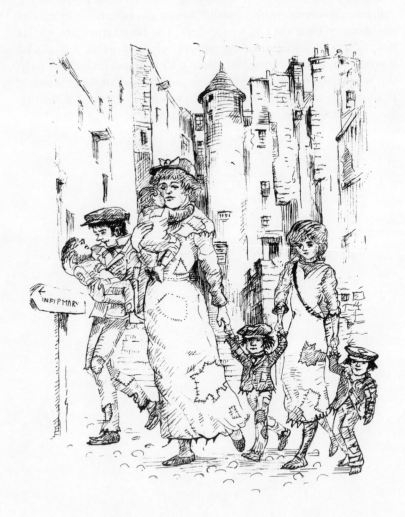

❧ 12 ❧

The Fever Epidemics

The doctor looked about my breast, and then about my back,
And then he shook his head and said, 'Your case looks very black.'
And first he sent me hot cayenne, and then gamboge to swallow,
But still my fever would not turn to scarlet or to yellow!

THOMAS HOOD

Thomas Hood recovered from his illness to write more of his cheerful poetry. Christine, Elizabeth, John, Alec, Hugh, Peter and David McDonald had less reason to be happy. Their home was in Blackfriars Wynd in Edinburgh and all seven were admitted to Edinburgh Royal Infirmary on the same day in February 1847. All were suffering from 'fever', the ward register calling it 'typhus'. Peter died.

Edinburgh experienced epidemics of 'fever' in 1843–4 and 1847–8, the huge increase in admissions to the Infirmary presenting problems for its managers. The problems were clinical, logistical, and financial. How these were dealt with is described here and in the next two chapters. In this chapter clinical cases are reported and the controversy about the diagnosis of the fever or fevers involved is briefly discussed.

There were so many admissions that one day at the end of 1847, a senior physician reported that ten patients admitted to his wards had died before his first ward round after their arrival. The board, worried about the large mortality (1,059 in 1847) explained that many patients had been brought to the Infirmary 'simply to die, many within forty-eight hours'. The high incidence of the disease in the insanitary Old Town can be seen from the following figures for 'fever' admissions that year:

New Town	203

Old Town:

1. Canongate and adjacent streets and closes	257
2. Cowgate and adjacent closes and wynds	866
3. Grassmarket and adjacent closes and wynds	734
4. High Street and adjacent closes and wynds	572

Rest of South Side	356

The clerical staff of the hospital managed, in spite of these numbers, to keep legible admission registers. The young doctors, who had to see everyone on admission, had difficulty in keeping up with the paperwork. Two of the actual ward journals from 1847 have survived. Instead of the usual long and careful admission notes, those on the 'fever' patients are brief, often scrawled, and often incomplete. Many were written by Dr Martin Lamb. The journal from which the following cases come is scuffed from frequent handling and contains a loose slip of paper with the notes of six other admissions in Lamb's writing. These were probably to be transcribed to the journal when he had time. The word 'synocha' used by Lamb correctly means 'any continuous fever' but was here used more loosely to mean simply a 'fever' case. The last case in the following list is from 1848 and the second journal.

MARY STEWART, aged 17
From Charity Workhouse.
19 May 1847. Admitted to ward. Patient was attacked with rigors eight days before admission. At present presents the usual appearances of synocha.

JESSIE MALCOLM, aged 12
St Mary's Wynd.
3 June 1847. Admitted to ward. Rigors two days before admission. Headache, eyes suffused. No eruption. Skin hot and dry.

JOHN CAMPBELL, aged 35
Irish. Now Crawford's Close. A labourer.
? July 1847. Admitted to ward. Shivered on Saturday having been perfectly well before. Rigors ever since. Headache and general

---

pains. No eruption. Eyes suffused. Râles chest. Shortly after admission conjunctiva became much more injected and typhoid [*sic*] stupor came on.[1]

℞ *Head blistered and stimulant continued.*

8 *July 1847.* Symptoms have assumed gradually a more typhoid character.

Turpentine enema

KATHY FLYNN, aged 32
Donegal. Now Bathgate.
6 August 1847. Admitted to ward. Shivered on the 1st.
11 *August 1847.* Has sweated a great deal last night and this morning feels somewhat relieved.

MARY FLYNN, aged 18 MONTHS
Donegal. Now Bathgate.
6 August 1847. She is the daughter of Kathy above. Admitted to ward suffering from smallpox.
18 August 1847. She died.

JEAN BROWN, aged 15
West Port.
6 A*ugust 1847.* Admitted to ward. Shivered on night of 31 July. Pulse 132. Skin pungently hot. Cough.[2]
9 August 1847. A measles eruption appeared in considerable abundance.
12 August 1847. Given wine since two days. Eruption somewhat receding.
17 August 1847. Improved since two days. Eruption disappeared. Has sweated to a considerable degree coincidentally with amelioration of symptoms. Pulse 104.

---

[1] This man's symptoms are not detailed but are probably due to typhus. The word 'typhoid' may mean 'typh-oid' or 'typhus-like', rather than 'typhoid' the disease. This ambiguity is to be found in much of the writing on these epidemics.

[2] Typhus causes patients to emit a strong odour, which may explain 'pungently'.

MARY THOMSON, aged 40
Leitrim. Now College Wynd.
6 August 1847. Admitted to ward. Shivered a week ago exactly.
Pulse 112. Measly eruption.
11 August 1847. Eyes suffused. Tenderness left groin. Eruption
abundant. Wine.
℞ *Hirudines 3 to anus.*[1]
12 August 1847. Tenderness in groin almost gone.
17 August 1847. Eruption blackens. Pulse 92. Cough troublesome.

ANNE LOUISE MCGINTY, aged 11
Cavan, now Cowgate
7 August 1847. Admitted to ward. No satisfactory account of
mode or time of attack. Pulse 141. Some mottling.
11 August 1847. Improved without diaphoresis.
17 August 1847. Dismissed cured.
Abstract: 'Typhus with mottling. Critical period unknown,
probably 14th or 15th day.'

KATE RILEY, aged 17
Armagh. Now Cowgate.
7 August 1847. Admitted to ward. Shivered on the 5th. General
pains. Has sweated a little every day since the attack. Pulse 141.
Lower part of legs of a bright, erythematous hue, disappearing on
pressure. Petechial spots on legs. Something like measly eruption
on thighs and hips. Skin hot and dry.
9 August 1847. Face has assumed almost the appearance of
Scarletina. Legs have become dingy where they were bright red.
Measly eruption doubtful. To have wine.
11 August 1847. Cough and oppression relieved. Redness of face
gone. Pulse 68.
2 September 1847. Dismissed cured.

---

[1] Three leeches were applied to the anus to treat the tenderness in the left
groin.

HELEN O'CONNOR, aged 22
Roscommon, Ireland. Now Canongate.
8 August 1847. Admitted to ward. Unable from stupor to answer questions. Great oppression. Eruption abundant. Said to have been ill upwards of two weeks.
17 August 1847. Pulse 82. Stupor in a great degree gone. Tongue cleans rapidly. Eruption indistinct; in some places 'tis [*sic*] converted into or replaced by small desquamating vesicles. Some abdominal tenderness.

MARGARET CAMERON, aged 52
George Square. A widow.
10 August 1847. Admitted to ward. Shivered a week ago exactly, having been perfectly well before. Raves a little. Pulse 128. Abundant measly eruption.
14 August 1847. Wine. Her purely asthenic symptoms have become well marked.
15 August 1847. 8 Died sinking [*sic*].

ROSIE TAYLOR, aged 40
Address? A married housewife
29 July 1848. Admitted to Ward 11. Four days ago, while sitting at a window, she was seized with a sense of coldness followed by severe shivering. In the evening she had severe headache followed by pain of back. Was not exposed to contagion of fever. Never had typhus.
   On examination expression typhoid [*sic*], skin hot, pulse 100, tongue furred, bowels confined.
℞ *To have a jalap and calomel purge and soda water for a drink.*
30 July 1848. Since last night she has had nearly constant muttering delirium. Can be roused at times.
℞ *Head to be shaved immediately.*[1] *To have six ounces of wine.*
31 July 1848. Pulse 110. Surface cold. Cannot be roused.
℞ *To have ten ounces of wine.*
1 August 1848. Died today at twelve noon.
Index of ward journal gives diagnosis as typhus.

---

[1] Shaving of the head was often done in patients with altered consciousness. It was followed by the application of cold soaks or a blistering agent.

BETTY BLACK, aged 8
Baillie's Court, Cowgate.
11 August 1847. Admitted to ward. No history obtainable. Measly eruption, mixed with darker spots impossible of reduction by pressure, which seem to be the 'nuclei' of the measly whorls. Skin hot and dry.
17 August 1847. Dismissed cured.
Abstract – typhus with eruption.

THE PROBLEM OF DIAGNOSIS

In the above case histories there are references to synocha, scarletina, typhus, typhus with mottling, typhus with eruption, typhoid, measles and smallpox. This illustrates how difficult it was for a doctor to know from which illnesses a patient was suffering, even when there might be many around him with similar symptoms. While the matter was academic in that no specific treatment was available, the precise diagnosis of the disease or diseases responsible for the Scottish epidemics in the 1840s was much discussed. The debate eventually centred on whether typhus and typhoid were one disease or two. The variablity of the terminology used confused the issue. Some talked of relapsing fever or the common epidemic fever; others of intermittent fever, or synocha, or even yellow fever. The following extracts from contemporary medical journals illustrate the main argument.

In 1840 a paper was published by Dr Alexander Stewart of Glasgow entitled 'Some observations on the nature and pathology of typhus and typhoid fever applied to the solution of the question of the identity or non-identity of the two diseases'. (*Edinburgh Medical Journal,* Vol. 55, 1840, p. 289)

Dr Christison, an Edinburgh physician, had his own views on 'fever' which he admitted were not shared by all and which were later criticised by William Tennant Gairdner. They were based on Christison's experience of past epidemics and, in passing, they provide a good story, retold in this book in the chapter headed 'One of the physicians'.

In 1842 the *Edinburgh Medical and Surgical Journal* published a review of an article by Elisha Bartlett, a professor of medicine in

Philadelphia, entitled 'A Review of Fever'. Bartlett held that 'all the recognised English works on fever are of little or no use to the American profession, either as a guide to a knowledge of the disease, or to the best means of cure. All work in the United Kingdom is not a sufficient or even safe guide for American practitioners and does not resemble the disease seen in the US.' Bartlett distinguished clearly between typhoid and typhus, including the lesions found in the Peyer's patches in the former. He adds that typhus is predominantly a disease of Ireland, Scotland and 'the northern British Empire', being rare in southern England, France and the United States. Describing them as 'radically dissimilar' his conclusion was that typhoid and typhus are different diseases.

The man who reviewed Bartlett's article was outraged. 'That the two diseases are essentially the same', he wrote, 'we cannot for a moment doubt, and the very fact mentioned so strongly by Dr Christison, and which we ourselves have frequently had occasion to verify, proves typhoid and typhus to be essentially the same disease; to be but simple variations of the same general epidemic.' The review goes on, 'Bartlett endeavours to show that typhoid and typhus have been by almost all confounded together, and that these British writings are useless as a guide to the practitioner'. It was, however, Bartlett who was right.

A Dr Smith of Glasgow agreed with Bartlett. Speaking in 1844 to the Glasgow University Medical Society on the 1842 Glasgow outbreak he said: 'Following as this epidemic did in the track of typhus fever, in the same location and spreading in similar manner, the opinion arose that these conditions were distanced only in some accidental occurrence. But most now think them different diseases'. [*Edinburgh Medical and Surgical Journal,* 62, 1844]

Professor F. A. E. Crew of Edinburgh claims that William Budd, also of Edinburgh, distinguished typhus from typhoid in 1843. (*Scientific Survey of South East Scotland,* British Association for the Advancement of Science, 1951)

In 1843 Dr Craigie published a paper entitled 'Notice of a febrile disorder which has prevailed at Edinburgh during the summer of 1843 [*Edinburgh Medical and Surgical Journal,* 59, 1843]. It comments: 'This febrile disorder is different from the typhus and synochus, the usual forms of continued fever in Edinburgh and neighbourhood. This is especially so as it is relapsing, there are no red spots as are found in typhus, it is not so productive of delirium as typhus, and finally the mortality is much lower than in typhus. 'But,' he goes on 'in some cases the rose-red spots of typhus [*sic*] were seen and, in some, an eruption of dark red or purple spots like purpura was seen in first attack alone.' Of 182 cases he reported relapses in 110. Some patients had 'faint jaundice'. He goes on 'unquestionably the distemper is unlike any febrile affection we have been in the habit of observing in this city. On the ninth of September, among 364 cases of fever in the Infirmary and the two fever sheds, 346 were cases of the epidemic and only 18 of genuine typhus'. He did not name this disease.

Professor William Henderson was a physician in the fever wards of the Infirmary and one of the first to use the microscope to study diseased organs. He was also one of the first to distinguish between typhus and the new epidemic fever seen in the 1844 epidemic. In an address to the Royal Medical Society of Edinburgh he begins by referring to the 'perplexity and confusion in which the whole subject of continued fever is so well known'. The object of his paper was 'to show that typhus fever and the epidemic fever of 1844 are essentially different diseases'. He dismissed the suggestion that the 1844 disease was 'only a milder form of typhus'. The first case Henderson saw in this epidemic was in February 1844 and he noted that 'it was widely different from any case previously seen. The first point that struck me as remarkable, and unlike what I had seen in typhus fever, was the faster pulse . . . ' (This suggests that the new disease was not typhoid where the pulse is slower than expected in relation to the temperature, not faster.)

Henderson does not name this disease. Nor did Craigie and nor did the minute of the Infirmary board of 11 March 1884 when it was decided that 'typhus and the common epidemic fever are to be separated in the wards'.

Finally William Tennant Gairdner, writing forty years after this debate, says that his views on fever differed from Professor Christison's both in 1840 and 1858. He concedes that the older man simply expressed the common classification of both Edinburgh and British physicians. 'Moreover at that time no other doctrine had been seriously entertained than that all the varieties of "continued fever" observed in these islands were merely varieties dependent upon the contemporary "epidemic constitution", they being in no repect specifically distinct from one another.' From the vantage point of

1882 Gairdner continues 'The progress of events, and especially microscopic pathology, has shown that synocha or relapsing fever is a worldwide disease e.g in India, Germany and this country, character- ised by a *spirillum* inhabiting the blood and identified with the fever and its successive relapses in the same individual, while it is of near absolute certainty that this organism is not found in typhus or any other disease except relapsing fever. The diseases in question are now commonly designated typhus, enteric, and relapsing fever.' Gairdner adds that, while he does not think so, there might just have been something in Christison's idea of the 'gradational' nature of these diseases, whereby they 'shade' into one another. This idea, he adds, was also held by other doctors who saw 'gradational merging' between scarletina, diphtheria and croup.

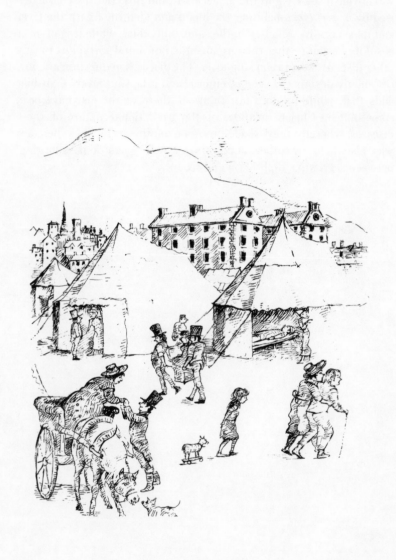

❧ 13 ❧

Logistical Problems of the Fever Epidemics

Is there any room at your head, Sanders?
Or any room at your feet?
Or any room at your twa sides
Where fain, fain I would sleep?

'Clerk Sanders' (old ballad)

The last chapter described the clinical aspects of the 1840s fever epidemics. This chapter looks at the problem the board faced in finding accommodation for such vast numbers of sick people. Much of the story is told in the words of the board's minutes. Apart from the first priority of finding beds, the dispersal of patients was affected by the current debate about the safest way to house people suffering from infectious illness. Was isolation a good idea? The size of the problem can be seen from the figures for total yearly admissions to the Royal Infirmary. The peaks of demand were in 1843–4 and 1847–8:

1840–3557	1844–5664	1847–7435
1841–3888	1845–3252	1848–7067
1842–3502	1846–3638	1849–3686
1843–4624		

Mid-1843. A shed had been erected in the Infirmary grounds to take the overflow from the wards. The generosity of the citizens of Edinburgh had allowed the small Surgeons' Square hospital to be reopened and it was now available to the managers for fever patients.
16 October 1843. The roof of the fever shed had blown down in a gale. Nobody had been hurt and everyone had been evacuated in half an hour. The builder replaced the roof at his own cost.
1 November 1843. A rota for doctors to care for the fever patients in the Surgeons' Square hospital had been put into operation.
11 March 1844. There was an inconclusive discussion as to whether

typhus cases and those suffering from 'the common epidemic fever' should be separated.

15 December 1845. Around this date there was much anxiety about the best way to manage fever cases. Two schools of thought existed. The first sought to mix such patients with general medical patients in the existing medical wards, the second to isolate them in fever wards. Some thought the second exposed the staff to too much risk from the 'concentrated atmosphere' of such wards. The apothecary's porter and 'the men who shaved the heads of the fever patients' had been affected with the disease during this year. Three apothecary's porters had acquired the disease in all, and this was felt to be an argument for distributing the cases around the medical wards.

Late December 1845. A different view was expressed by Dr Robertson, one of the Infirmary physicians. In a letter to the board he wrote: 'The fever has been mild, and the small amount of it observed in the usual hotbeds of the Old Town, coupled with the fact that in the fever wards of the Infirmary the attendants have escaped infection, shows that its contagious properties are less virulent. I refrain from speculating on what might happen if a more contagious epidemic prevailed. Our first duty is to the sick, and their interest would be better served with a system of roomy and well-ventilated fever wards, rather than continuing with the experiment [of mixing fever and general patients]'.

This was the final decision but it did not happen immediately. The number of fever cases occurring in the general wards was considered at each board meeting for many months before a decision was reached.

3 January 1846. The annual report noted that the funds of the hospital had improved and 'under providence there has been comparatively little fever and a material abatement of disease generally among the poorer classes. But a continuance of this state of things cannot be calculated upon . . . '

16 February 1846. The experiment on the distribution in the wards of fever patients continued. Erysipelas was also frequent and ward 18 was shortly to be opened for male erysipelas cases.

19 April 1847. A new problem arose. On the 12th of this month, ninety-three railway labourers were in the Infirmary with fever, scurvy and other illnesses and injuries. 'The large wooden shed is to be opened to accommodate patients with scurvy.'

20 April 1847. The mattress shed was now in use for patients as the hospital was full of fever cases.

24 May 1847. Four tents from the Castle were put up, more being available if needed. Iron bedsteads came 'from Leith' [*sic*]. Twill cotton sheeting at 40 inches wide, and English blankets at 9/3 d. a pair, were bought for fifty patients.

14 June 1847. The tent at Archers' Hall was now in use and a shed was being built which would be ready in two weeks. The garrets were being cleared for patients and the Chapel was in use as a ward.

21 June 1847. It was discussed carefully whether the parochial boards of the city and of St Cuthbert's should be asked for temporary accommodation for convalescent patients. The city responded quickly and favourably.

5 July 1847. Dr Coldstream had taken charge of the fever patients in the fever shed and in the east garret. No extra physician was to be appointed.

12 July 1847. A petition was received from several inhabitants of Surgeons' Square complaining of the opening of a convalescent house for fever patients in close contact with their dwellings. They were told this had nothing to do with the Infirmary.

26 July 1847. 'The young gentleman presently acting as physician's non-resident clerk in the fever shed and the tents, and giving great satisfaction to the physician, would be willing to remain in the town during autumn provided he could be accommodated in the Royal Infirmary.' This was agreed.

1 November 1847. The chapel was now 'empty, cleaned and back to usual function.'

4 April 1848. A fever shed was taken down.

Mid-1848. The Surgeons' Square hospital was closed.

6 October 1848. 'Two cases, having all the symptoms of Asiatic cholera' had been brought to the Royal the previous day, and both had died. It was decided to keep wards 7 and 17 as male and female cholera wards if more cases came in immediately, but otherwise to arrange for the Surgeons' Square hospital – 'formerly used as a fever hospital' – to be reopened to take all cases. It was to be under the control of the city parochial board.

6 November 1848. Dr Martin Lamb resigned as clerk in the Royal having been appointed by the parochial board as resident medical officer in the cholera hospital.

1 January 1849. The annual report showed that, by today and as a result of the sharp fall in fever cases, four fever sheds had been taken down and Thomson's House had closed. The fever hospital in Surgeons' Square and the Infirmary's ward 17, a fever ward, had also closed [although the fever hospital had reopened when cholera arrived in the city]. The board 'was glad to see the closure of rough and ready accommodation in garrets, tents and sheds.'

5 February 1849. A deputation from the city parochial board was seen. The Infirmary board agreed to take back control of the fever (now cholera) hospital as cholera cases were much diminished and there had been no new ones for several days.

26 March 1849. Cholera hospital closed as there had been no cases for two weeks. This hospital was finally shut at the end of 1849.

Edinburgh Royal Infirmary had coped successfully with both the clinical and the logistical demands of the epidemics. How well it coped with the rise in the need for finance will be seen in the next chapter.

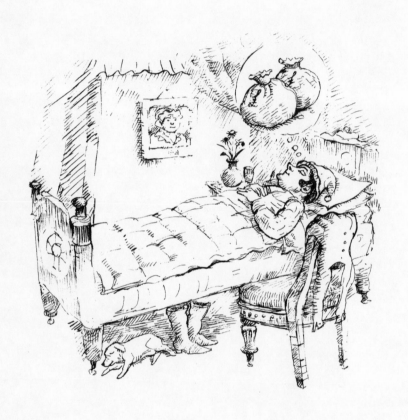

❧ 14 ❧

Funding the Infirmary in the Fever Years

For I did dream of money-bags tonight.

SHAKESPEARE, *The Merchant of Venice* 2,5,17

Shylock's dream would have been well understood by the hard-pressed treasurer of the Infirmary board during the 1840s. Not only did he have to depend on voluntary contributions to cover the normal costs of running the Infirmary but this was the decade of Edinburgh's two major fever epidemics. The huge increase in the number of patients meant a corresponding need for more money to provide for them. Opened to care for the sick of Edinburgh and district, the Infirmary could reasonably expect financial support from that community. This had been generously given but now, in the peak fever years of 1843–4 and 1847–8, the treasurer had two problems. The first was the sudden serious fall in the steady income from the Established Church which followed the Disruption. Although steps were taken to correct this, there were times when the Infirmary's income was dangerously low. The second problem for the treasurer was caused by the prolonged failure of the Irish potato harvests. As a result, Edinburgh's population had been greatly increased by Irish families, in the city in search of work. Their poor housing meant that they were more likely to become fever victims and require hospital care. The Infirmary's admission figures prove this. In 1848, for example, the figures were:

Scots	4,155 of whom 2,175 were fever cases.	
Irish	2,563 of whom 1,915 were fever cases.	
English	237	
Others	109	

The board could not refuse to admit ill patients but noted that the Irish 'had the advantage of medical care by means of the benevolent contributions of the inhabitants of this town'. The cost of a 'fever' admission was estimated at 30 shillings per patient. An 'Irish total' was calculated, to be used if eventually the board felt forced to ask the government for financial help. board members did not want to make such an appeal.

The following information comes from the board minutes and shows just how successfully the treasurer, the board and the people of Edinburgh solved the problem. It must have been particularly satisfying for them to record at the end of the decade that, in that year (1849), the Infirmary's income had exceeded its expenditure for the first time in many years.

4 January 1841. It was felt that, this being a hospital dependent on voluntary funding, insufficient support was being received from the public, especially 'as the high character of the medical attendants was bringing patients from the most distant parts of the kingdom'.

8 January 1841. The 'watching department' of the police gave £15 to Infirmary funds; the fire department £3 14*s.*

6 September 1841. £43 received from workers on the Craigton branch of the Edinburgh and Glasgow Railway.

31 July 1843. A public meeting was held in the Assembly Rooms, under the Lord Provost's chairmanship, to boost income for the Royal Infirmary in the fever outbreak. The city was to be divided into districts and every house visited to extract money. This allowed the reopening of the Surgeons' Square hospital for fever cases.

11 October 1843. The newspaper carried thanks to the population but emphasised that more money was required and was to be directly collected.

1 November 1843. The second public collection took place. Mitchell, who owned a grocer's business in Shakespeare Square, donated a cask of arrowroot to the Infirmary.

31 March 1845. Approval was given to a request from the House Committee asking 'if some old silver plate, not now used at Matron's table, could be sold for Infirmary funds.'

17 November 1845. A letter was sent to the directors of the North British Railway Company calling their attention to the number of accidents and other cases involving people in their employment and soliciting a subscription to the funds of the hospital.

3 January 1846. The annual report noted that funds were at a better level than for some years past. This was attributed to various causes including more donations and larger legacies. There had also been fewer patients in 1845. The report included the passage 'The past year [in Edinburgh] has been one of almost unexampled prosperity. There has been full employment for the labouring classes while provisions have been abundant and at reasonable prices and hence, under providence, there has been comparatively little fever and a material abatement of disease generally among the poorer classes. But a continuance of this state of things cannot be calculated upon.'

Those auditing the Infirmary accounts for 1845 added a note to their financial report saying they had found that 'a salutary control and effective discipline had, under a spirit of kindness, been exercised over all the officers of the institution'.

Salaries for 1846 were determined. They included matron £80, cupper £21, chaplain £50 and precentor £5 5s.

22 June. Edinburgh and Glasgow Railway donated £5 5s. to Infirmary funds.

21 September. In response to requests for funds the following donations were received:

1. From an anonymous donor, 9/6d. in postage stamps [introduced in 1840].
2. James Russell of Edinburgh gave £150 on condition that the Infirmary would pay him an annuity of £6 for life. This was agreed.
3. £3 5s.1¾d. from boys and girls of Heriot's School, High School Yards.
4. £2 5s. from a shopkeeper, 'being money left in his shop, less the expenses of advertising.'
5. Ten bottles of port and one of sherry from session of St Andrew's Church.

21 June 1847. St Cuthbert's parochial board donated £80 after being approached, and Edinburgh churches gave extra funding. Charles Dick, brewer, gave twenty hogsheads of beer for patients, and an anonymous donor gave 'twelve dozen of port wine – this to be put in the newspapers.'

3 January 1848. The parochial boards of the county had not, it was felt, fully paid what they ought and they were reminded that 'Edinburgh Royal Infirmary has always afforded relief to the sick and hurt among the labouring classes on a more liberal footing than any similar institution'.

April 1848. A suggestion was made to the board, from a member of the public, that Miss Jenny Lind be asked to sing for the Infirmary's funds. The suggestion was turned down.

19 June 1848. Edinburgh and district parochial boards to be charged 9*d.* per day for the care of their pauper patients.

26 June 1848. Kirknewton's Inspector of the Poor had received a bill from Edinburgh Royal for care given to his pauper patients. He wrote asking if it could be 'departed from' as a collection for the funds of the Infirmary, which was about to start in his area, might be 'injured'. His request was refused.

11 October 1848. The Infirmary had installed a charity box within the hospital. At this meeting it was decided that donations to it might be increased by having it moved from the main staircase to the outer gate.

2 November 1848. The Parochial Board of St Cuthbert's offered 9*d.* per day if Edinburgh Royal would take their cholera patients. They were told that Edinburgh Royal had resolved not to take cholera patients. St Cuthbert's were thus left to send their cases to Surgeons' Square hospital which they did not want to do as the city Parochial Board was to run it.

1 January 1849. The annual report noted that the board was 'again faced with an increased financial burden due to the great numbers of the vagrant Irish being treated'. It was suggested that the government be asked to help. The hospital was at that point so crowded that patients were being housed in the chapel, the garrets and even tents in the grounds. The report comments 'No man who has the slightest spark of humanity in his breast but must be appalled at such a state of matters being allowed to exist in the metropolis of Scotland, and that, too, at a time when philanthropy is so distinguished a feature of the age'.

The report goes on to suggest that the working class trades might form auxiliary societies to raise contributions for their hospital costs and an Address should be circulated to the trades to this effect. In 1847, for example there had been admitted 35 bakers, 21 cabinet makers, 47 carpenters and joiners, 32 carters, 27 coachmen, 96 dressmakers, 63 farm servants and field workers, 41 gardeners, 58 hawkers, 2,379 labourers, 41 masons, 557 servants, 166 shoemakers, 130 tailors and 'many others unnecessary to be detailed'.

Furthermore, in 1846, patients had been seen from twenty-eight Scottish counties other than Edinburgh, while contributions to the Infirmary were received from just five. 'Many non-contributors' it was noted, 'are enjoying the benefit of the immense Highland destitution fund.' It was felt, therefore, that 'this fund should defray Highland patients' costs'.

It was pointed out, again in the annual report, that the proprietors of coal works marketing their coal in Glasgow, 'gratuitously furnished' Glasgow Royal Infirmary with coal. Perhaps those Proprietors marketing their coal in Edinburgh could be asked to do likewise?

It was suggested that the government might free the wine used in patients' care from duty. This would save £300 per annum.

Finally the annual report noted two further donations. Linen from St James's Palace, London had been gifted to the Infirmary (per Lord Breadalbane), and Nelson, the publishers, had gifted thirty-eight volumes.

12 March 1849. £78 11*s.* was received from officers of the Edinburgh Garrison, being the surplus from theatrical performances at the Theatre Royal on 2nd inst. The minutes noted 'the handsome conduct of the officers of the garrison towards this charity was admirable, and the donation accepted with the grateful thanks of the board.'

26 March 1849. Aberdeen Royal Infirmary asked if Edinburgh Royal had received any money from the government for its fever cases. It had not.

3 April 1849. The cashier of the Edinburgh and Bathgate Railway wrote to say men working on that railway were to contribute to the Infirmary and would like to know if, should any of them require admission, their donations would be used to defray their own expenses. This was agreed.

In conclusion the board's treasurer was able to report to his colleagues that, as that December drew to a close, the Infirmary's 1849 income had exceeded its expenditure for the first time in many years. This had been achieved without government help. An important cause of the improvement was the increased income from newly organised workers' trade groups.

So the treasurer could sleep more peacefully in his bed on these wintry December nights. If, like Shylock, he still dreamt of money-bags, at least they were now comfortably full.

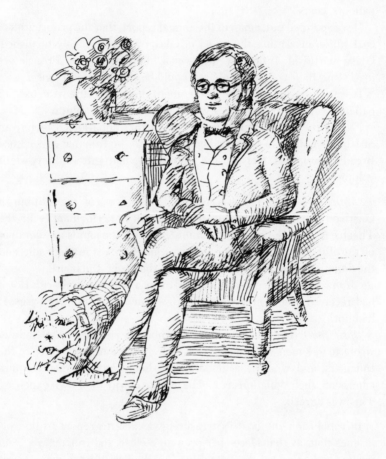

❧ 15 ❧

W. T. Gairdner, Pathologist and Physician

His words of learned length, and thund'ring sound
Amazed the gazing rustic ranged around,
And still they gazed and still the wonder grew
That one small head could carry all he knew.

OLIVER GOLDSMITH, 1770

William Tennant Gairdner was one of those men whose intellectual capacity is in a different league from ordinary mortals. This was recognised early. All the comments on him in his junior years were favourable, his tenure of a clerkship was extended on his request and he had no trouble in being appointed to the jobs he wanted on the Infirmary staff. He did blot his copybook once, however, when the board reprimanded him for being out of the hospital twice after hours in the same week. He progressed rapidly from clerk to Infirmary pathologist to physician. His last appointment was to the Chair of Medicine in Glasgow University. While there he received a knighthood. His reputation as a physician was equal to that of Robert Syme in surgery.

Ian Craig's case record was written by Gairdner. It shows his unique, lawyer-like style, the patient's history and physical signs being clearly described:

IAN CRAIG, aged 36
High Street. A baker.
31 May 1845. Admitted to the Infirmary. He states that he is a Scotsman by birth and education but has been ten years at London engaged in his trade of a baker. During his residence there, as well as during his former residence in Scotland, he says that he has enjoyed good health generally; that he has passed through scarlet fever, measles and typhus many years ago with-

---

out any impression being made upon his general health; that from the nature of his occupation he has been exposed to alterations of temperature without any bad consequences resulting; and that his constitution remained unbroken until four years ago when he had rheumatic fever which disappeared, but since that period he considers himself more liable to suffer from cold. In May 1844 he was confined to bed with a cough which was accompanied by rigors and sweating and he became reduced in strength so as to be unable to return to his employment.

On examination emaciated, face pale with a slight hectic flush. Frequent short cough, shortness of breath, cold night sweats, haemoptysis. Loud bronchophony and gurgling râles and dullness on percussion below left clavicle. Can only walk on level ground. Appetite good.'

The diagnosis was phthisis.

Gairdner's description of the clinical signs in another case of tuberculosis, a miner from Airdrie called Joseph Connarty, was equally clear. He wrote : 'There is dullness on percussion under both clavicles. Loud bronchophony between the second and third ribs on the left side above the nipple. Respiratory murmur rough and hollow below left clavicle. Heart sounds and action natural. Pulse 112. Has at present cephalalgia. There is great weakness and extreme emaciation. Expression anxious; pallor of face.'

GAIRDNER AS PATHOLOGIST

This ability to record facts clearly probably helped when he applied for the post of pathologist to the Infirmary in 1848. He became responsible for the Edinburgh Pathology Register, a series of large leather-bound notebooks in which the findings at every post-mortem examination were recorded. He wrote almost all of these himself in great detail. On the fly-leaf of one volume he noted that, if he had to be away from the hospital, he tried later to discuss each examination with his deputy. When it did fall to a deputy to write a report, some of Gairdner's marginal additions are blunt. The case of Williamina McCann includes a short but typically precise report by Gairdner on the post-mortem. The clinical history here was written by John Struthers, a member of a well-known Edinburgh Royal Infirmary medical 'dynasty'.

WILLIAMINA MCCANN, aged 55
2 Fleshmarket Close. Married.
10 January 1849. Admitted to ward 11. Her friend, who lives on the same floor, states that on New Year's night Wales and her husband left home to see a friend in the West Port. The person has not a home, and they walked about for about two hours when Wales began to complain of the cold. She and her husband entered a spirit shop and had a glass of spirits each. On leaving the shop she spoke a single word and then fell over on to her left side, attempting to support herself by the railing. She was insensible. She lay a short time in a common stair and was then removed by the Police to the station house where she was kept during the night. Was taken home next morning in the same insensible state.

From this up to the 4th she lay quite still in bed. Asked for nothing but on being shaken, or spoken to loudly, spoke a little and answered questions but could not recognise individuals or at least could not pronounce their names. The eyes remained closed. There was no twisting of the face. The left arm and leg were completely paralysed.

On Thursday the 4th she became delirious and continued raving until the 7th when it became less. The delirium was not furious; she was constantly talking but had no convulsions, nor did she give sudden cries or starts. On the 8th, two days ago, she remained drowsy. Asked for a glass of whisky – got some tea.

On admission face hands and feet cold and blue; at first sight she has the appearance of one in the collapsed stage of cholera. The face is covered with a cold moisture. Pupils contracted, both equally. They are insensible to light. Cannot be roused by pinching, loud talking or by injecting water into the ears.

Pulse 100. Breath rapid with tracheal râles. Right arm and leg, on being pinched, are slightly moved. Left arm and leg completely paralysed. Left side of face is completely insensible. No twisting of face. No scalp injury or depression of the cranium.
℞ *Oleum Crotonis gtt: 2.*[1]

---

[1] Croton oil was used as a purgative. It was placed on the tongue of unconscious patients. Being very toxic and irritant it was administered in a dose of so many drops (*guttae*).

℞ *Mass: pilul: colocynth. Sumat statim et hora somni 1 pilula.*[1]
To have a large mustard poultice applied to each leg.
11 January 1849. Continues in much the same state. Bowels not moved.
℞ *Oleum Crotonis gtt: 4*
To have a piece of lint 3" square dipped in strong aquae ammonia and applied to vertex.
12 January 1849. No blister formed on scalp though ammonia was applied for ½ hour. Pulse almost imperceptible. Surface cold and covered with clammy moisture. She is evidently moribund.
12 January 1849 (vespere).[2] She died an hour after visit without anything remarkable occurring.
Sectio Cadaveris
The posterior half of the right lateral ventricle is occupied by a blood clot, which also infiltrates the cerebral substance to the depth of several lines. Beyond this, for half an inch or so, the cerebral substance is softened and slightly discoloured. The foramen of Munro is dilated so as to admit a goose quill.[3]

---

[1] Colocynth was probably used here as another purgative; two were often given together. It may however, have been given for another indication listed in Beasley, namely 'as a revulsive in affections of the brain'. A 'revulsive' was defined as a counterirritant, or a means of using a substance to act on one disordered organ by its effect on another.

[2] 'Vespere' means 'in the evening'.

[3] A 'line' was a unit of measurement equivalent to one twelfth of an inch.

TEACHER AND PHYSICIAN

Gairdner enjoyed teaching and was popular with his students. On becoming pathologist, for example, he wrote immediately to the board to ask permission to give voluntary Saturday morning lectures on pathological topics. This was granted and the lectures were immediately fully subscribed. The board also agreed to his request to give a quarterly lecture to students entitled 'New facts and inquiries in pathological anatomy'.

His capacity for hard work was reflected in the large number of articles and papers he wrote and presented. He was not afraid to be honest. In an obituary on Sir Robert Christison, for example, Gairdner uncompromisingly dismissed the latter's ideas on the nature of the fever or fevers responsible for the 1840s epidemics in Scotland.

Footnote on the 'Stewart watercolours'

In the early 1990s sixty-three original watercolours, depicting a series of pathological specimens, were discovered in a storeroom in Dundee University. All were signed by the same artist, Neil Stewart. They were all dated around 1850. How they came to be in Dundee was a mystery, the solution to which is to be found in an article in the *Lancet* of 5 September 1998. All that need be said here is that William Tennant Gairdner was involved!

UNUSUAL CASES FROM THE JOURNALS: III

SUSAN BRUCE, aged 20
Queensferry. A servant.
28 April 1841. Admitted to surgical wards of Professor Syme.

Admitted on account of ulceration on the sole of the left foot at the root of the little toe. She was a patient here for the same disease in January last. It was then looked upon as a case of mercurio-venereal sore and was treated accordingly with the black wash[1] and hydriodide of potash[2] with the effect of completely curing the disease though after a long lapse in time. She says that she has not been living irregularly since she was dismissed and that the sore reappeared after a long day's journey on foot.

This explanation is improbable.

To be put on the same plan of treatment as formerly. The sore is exactly the same as it was at first.

2 May 1841. Under the use of the black wash externally and the hydriodide of potash internally the sore has greatly diminished in size.

24 May 1841. Dismissed cured.

MOLLY STEVENSON, aged 13 MONTHS
Address not known
31 July 1844. Admitted to surgical wards of Professor Syme.

This child was born with both feet in the condition usually denominated as Talipes Varus, the toes being turned inwards and the heels upwards.

3 August 1844. The tendo achilles and the tendon of the tibialis anterior were today divided on both feet.

9 August 1844. Dismissed cured.   M. C.

[1] 'Black Wash' (also known as lotio hydrargyri nigra or black mercurial lotion) was a lotion in which hydrarg. chlor. or calomel (known also in Edinburgh and Dublin as calomelas) was mixed with aquae calcis (liquor calcis or lime water). It was to be applied to 'indolent and venereal sores' according to a Dr Hooper, quoted by Beasley.

[2] Hydriodide of potassium- here in a dose of one scruple (20 grains) in water- was said by Beasley 'to exert an almost specific effect over scrofulus disorders, and the various symptoms of secondary syphilis'.

CAMERON MCLEAN, aged 2½

Todderick's Wynd[1]

26 August 1844. Admitted to surgical wards of Professor Syme.

26 August 1844. About three months ago this child was observed to become more peevish and irritable than usual. The calls to micturate shortly after became frequent . These symptoms in the course of time became more aggravated and a fortnight before admission prolapsus ani supervened.

A sound introduced into the bladder detects the presence of a stone. There is no blood found in the urine. The calls to micturate are now constant so that it is impossible to keep the patient dry. The gut is almost constantly prolapsed.

29 August 1844. The operation of lithotomy was today performed and a stone consisting of lithic acid and the size and shape of a large nut extracted.[2]

30 August 1844. He has passed a good night and seems in all respects doing well.

6 September 1844. Since last night he has had an attack of diarrhoea for which Mist: Creta[3] was prescribed and his bowels are again in good order. He has cried a good deal on account of his mother's absence but his condition remains favourable.

8 September 1844. His mother, being unable to attend to him in the House [*i.e.* in hospital], has been allowed to take him home. He continues to do well. Dismissed cured.

[1] Todderick's Wynd, which ran between the Cowgate and the High Street, was one of the narrower and dirtier alleys of Edinburgh's Old Town. In 1851 an anonymous writer in a pamphlet entitled 'An Inquiry into Destitution, Prostitution and Crime in Edinburgh', describing one family's home in this squalid and notorious wynd. 'A cellar, for it was nothing else, and a very small one too, was inhabited by a man, his wife and their infant child. Furniture there was absolutely none. A bundle of straw on the damp and earthen floor served for their bed; and the fire, and it was a mere spark, was on the hearthstone. The aspect was most desolate and it had a chill earthy smell that made one shudder on entering. The features of the whole three, even of the infant, had that pinched look that so tells of hunger – their eyes were sunken and the facial bones were keenly and unduly prominent'.

[2] Lithic acid is an old name for uric acid.

[3] 'Mist: Creta' is Chalk Mixture.

ANDREW CALDER, aged 36
Chirnside. A labourer.
11 July 1844. Admitted to surgical wards of Professor Syme.

Eight weeks ago, while cutting out a portion of the nail of the right great toe which was growing into the flesh, he injured the matrix and drew a little blood. He took no notice of this for three or four days when he observed that the affected foot was weak and the seat of uneasy sensations which shot up the leg. The weakness has since continue to increase in spite of leeches and blisters applied to the foot and he is now subject to pain over the whole body.

Nothing is found on examining the part but he is unable to walk. He has a weak sickly appearance and his pulse is quite full and bounding.

To have hot baths and Dover's powders.

17 July 1844. He expresses a determination to return home and, though strongly advised to remain, he peremptorily refuses and is accordingly dismissed.

K. K.

The admission register gives the diagnosis as – nervous excitement.

RICHARD DAVIDSON, aged 24
Greenock. A painter.
3 March 1841. Admitted to surgical wards of Professor Syme. He is a painter and has been engaged in painting devices on boards (in which he chiefly employs white lead) for the last three years. Neither he nor any of his fellow workmen have been affected with colic.

Six months ago he first noticed a weakness in his right shoulder. At the same time the joint was the subject of a dull rheumatic pain, also felt in the sole and great toe of the right foot. The weakness of the arm has increased and in the past one month he has lost all power of the deltoid muscle. Has lately developed the same sort of pain in the left hip but there is no weakness of this joint.

On examination the inner side of the right foot and great toe are swollen and painful on pressure. These parts appear oedematous but do not pit on pressure. The right deltoid is wasted and not above one half the size of its fellow. Patient appears emaciated and a great part of the body is covered by a scaly eruption.

Leeches, blisters, poultices and cataplasms have been at various times employed. He has also had various internal remedies but without effect.

Bowels to be regulated. To have a warm bath nightly.

℞ *Pulv: Rhei:* 1 drachm.[1] *Carb: Sodae:* 2 drachms. *Misce et divide in pulv: 6. Sumat unum bis in die*

14 March 1841. A blister to the affected shoulder. No improvement has yet taken place.

27th Aug Blister to the leg and repeated shocks from the electrical machine have been employed but without improvement. He was today sent to the medical clinical wards.[2]

ANN MURPHY, aged 17

Steven Law's Close. A pedlar.

Admitted ? date. States that she left County Leitrim, Ireland at fourteen years of age previous to which she had no particular employment and enjoyed good health. Her diet seems to have been somewhat better than the class of Irish generally to which she belongs, namely to breakfast potatoes, bread or porridge, always with milk; to dinner generally the same with fish or ham about once a week but seldom soup or fresh beef. Seldom any meal taken between dinner at 2 pm and supper at 8 pm when the same fare was again taken.

After leaving Ireland she came direct to Edinburgh and has since lived in a confined close in the Cowgate during which her diet has consisted of bread and tea to breakfast, frequently beef to dinner – if not, tea and dry bread – with potatoes and porridge to

---

[1] The rhubarb and carbonate of soda were to be mixed and divided into six powders of which one was to be taken twice daily. Rhei (rhubarb) which had 'almost infinite uses' (Beasley) was here used as a purgative. Beasley says that 'the species of rhubarb called Turkey rhubarb is the best in quality. It is obtained, through Russia, from some part of the Chinese Empire'.

[2] 'The electrical machine' produced a galvanic current by chemical action.

supper. By trade she travelled about the neighbourhood selling small wares but was seldom exposed to wet or cold.

Two years ago was attacked with haemoptysis, unaccompanied by cough and expectoration, recurring regularly about once a week for six months after which it disappeared. Her health continued unimpaired for a year but when out selling her goods she got cold and wet and almost immediately began to complain of cough and much expectoration. This has never left her, her health gradually giving way and her strength failing so that two weeks ago she had to stop work and has been confined to bed ever since. No member of her family has ever been known to suffer from pulmonary disease.

On examination extremely week and emaciated, the whole surface cold and livid. There are creps and râles throughout. The heart is of unnatural size with cardiac dullness to right of sternum. There is a blowing systolic murmur at the apex.

11 Novemeber. While getting into bed at ten a.m. she suddenly dropped down as if in a fit. She was immediately lifted into bed, the chest heaved convulsively, the veins of the neck and face became greatly distended, the whole surface livid and she expired in about three minutes.

Sectio Cadaveris

Heart enlarged. Enormously dilated right ventricle and auricle. The right ventricle forms the apex, its walls ½ inch thick. Tricuspid orifice wide. Valve of pulmonary artery healthy. Left ventricle normal; left auricle dilated. Mitral orifice admitted only point of little finger, its lips united for about two thirds of the extent. No atheroma on valve but edges thickened. Aortic valves thickened. Lungs show phthisis and much emphysema.[1]

Diagnosis in ward journal – bronchitis. Phthisis. Morbus cordis.

---

[1] The post-mortem examination shows the classical appearances of mitral stenosis as well as pulmonary tuberculosis. There were thus two possible causes for the haemoptysis.

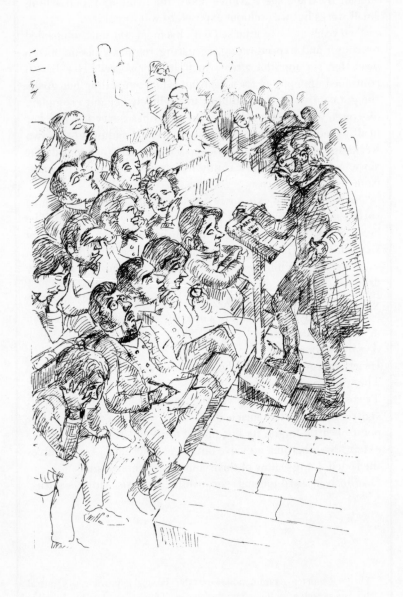

❦ 16 ❦

Edinburgh and the Medical Press

All newspaper and journalistic activity is an intellectual
brothel from which there is no retreat.

L. TOLSTOY, 1871

The *Lancet* and the *Edinburgh Medical Journal* in the 1840s shared the
same blunt style. They exercised this in leading articles, random
news paragraphs and in their correspondence pages. The *Lancet* was
well-informed and frank on the medical politics of Edinburgh. The
Edinburgh Medical Journal was just as uninhibited in its comments on
medical personalities in the city. The following illustrations of their
style begin with the case of Dr J. R. Cormack.

Dr Craigie, one of the Infirmary physicians, was to be on leave of
absence for six months. Dr Cormack, a junior ordinary physician who
was deputising, asked if he could give lectures as part of his new
responsibilities. He was told by the board that this was not required
as one of the other senior physicians would be giving Craigie's
lectures. Dr Cormack was not pleased. He wrote to the board from
131 Princes Street as follows:

> I have given your letter my most careful consideration. As there is
> a determination on your part to prevent me from participating in
> any of the advantages fairly belonging the responsible, laborious
> and personally hazardous office of Infirmary Physician, I feel that
> I should be wanting in self-respect as well as in duty to my family
> did I any longer retain the appointment. I now therefore resign it
> into your hands.   (Signed) J. R. Cormack.

He received an uncompromising reply. The resignation was accepted and it was explained that Cormack's letter was written under a
misconception as to the managers' intentions. He was thanked for his
past service.

Confrontations like this were meat and drink to the *Lancet*. It published this correspondence, presumably having received it from Cormack, and also a long editorial on the subject. This included the following passage. 'The extraordinary conduct of the managers of the Royal Infirmary of Edinburgh with regard to Dr J. R. Cormack's request to give instruction to pupils who follow him in his visits, reveals the state of blind, narrow-minded ignorance of the true interests of patients and medical science which we should scarcely have credited on the part of public functionaries in northern Athens had it not been so clearly proven. He should have been warmly thanked instead of being flatly and uncourteously denied his request.'

Others agreed. Among the letters the *Lancet* received was one from 'A friend of the sick poor' published on 17 November 1845. This concluded 'As a fitting sequel to your recent exposure of the conduct of the managers of Royal Infirmary of Edinburgh, I think you ought to state in the *Lancet* that these reckless officials have appointed as Dr Cormack's successor a gentleman aged, at the utmost, twenty-five. This is Dr Robertson, the youngest man in the College of Physicians. The rejected candidates were Dr Andrew, Dr Hughes Bennett and Dr MacKellar, all graduates in medicine before Robertson left school. I hope the citizens of Edinburgh will bestir themselves to reform their Infirmary and until that is done they ought to withhold their contributions. Men of experience, and not boys, ought to be hospital physicians. But of course practitioners of standing would require to be treated with some consideration, and that would not suit.'

HOMEOPATHY

Homeopathy was too much for the *Lancet*'s sense of what was acceptable in British medicine. In an editorial of 9 January 1847 it remarked 'Professor Henderson [of Edinburgh] should be removed from office as he believes in homeopathy. The English universities are said to be slow in reform but now the Alma Mater of the Monroes, the Cullens and the Gregories seems even more indolent. The number of students will fall off . . . as news gets round that such professional laxity is tolerated. With homeopathic teachers, they may depend upon it, the classes will soon be infinitesimal.'

The editorial goes on to suggest that 'everyone memorialises the town council, the appointing body. It is preposterous to found a practice of medicine and healing of diseases upon doses of simple medicaments so attenuated that a single grain would supply the entire population of the globe in all diseases for many generations. The drugs for four hundred million people for a whole century might be readily carried over the world in the nutshell carriage of Queen Mab.'

THE RELIGIOUS TESTS AND SYME

Nor did the *Lancet* approve of the religious 'tests' applied in appointing Edinburgh University professors. These required that appointees must be members of 'that branch of the Scottish Protestant church presently favoured by the state'. A letter of 20 May 1848, signed 'MD Edinae', protests against their proposed reimposition. The fact that the tests 'have been probably illegally in abeyance for fifty years' has, the writer feels, 'been of benefit to the good reputation of Edinburgh'. He concludes his letter by stating that reintroduction would be disadvantageous and adds that Syme would not have been appointed if the tests had not been ignored earlier. The same correspondent would have welcomed the *Lancet*'s editorial in July that year in which it was noted that 'the religious tests applied in the appointment of Professors at Edinburgh University by the town council are now to be abandoned'.' The *Lancet* welcomed this repeal of 'a last remnant of religious persecution'.

It had previously referred to the matter obliquely, when noting that Mr Syme had been invited to a public dinner prior to taking up the chair of surgery at St Thomas's Hospital in London. The journal noted 'He accepted the invitation [to the dinner] and on that day he will be prepared to receive the congratulations, solaces and lamentations of his professional brethren. It will be gratifying to the friends of religious freedom to learn that a 'pagan' is to be vice-president of this assembly of learned men!'

The *Lancet*, often wry, was not above sarcasm. Syme did not like London and remained there for only a short time before returning to his old job in Edinburgh. The *Lancet* said 'the statement and counterstatement, rumour and counter-rumour regarding Mr Syme's return to Edinburgh appear now to be definitely at rest. We are glad to be able to say so, and his friends may congratulate the "new" professor on being once more firmly seated amongst them. We trust for his own sake we shall not have to issue a bulletin to the contrary next week'.

A LETTER FROM 'VERAX'

It was not only the editorials that reverberated around the medical establishment of Edinburgh. The *Lancet's* correspondence columns were equally lively. The doctor who hid behind the name 'Verax' sounded upset.

The journal had published a letter which claimed that some new Edinburgh graduates were 'grossly ignorant'. 'Verax' responded on 3 February 1849: 'This is too true. The present system of giving medical degrees to beardless striplings is proving ruinous to the profession. Many new graduates start in country towns and villages and are full of self-confidence, trying to overawe [others]'. He goes on to list three examples of the lack of literacy of one new Edinburgh graduate:

1. To medicines and attendance on wife on 10th and 11th Jully.
2. Sir, please give the bearer of this two ounces of the milk of sulphur and you will oblidge me.
3. Please to fill this vial with paregoric [a camphorated tincture of opium] 10 gr. turbeth mineral.

'Verax' then comments on the same young doctor's clinical skills, listing first a medical patient and then two maternity cases:

1. This learned doctor bled an elderly delicate anaemic woman to fatal syncope! She expired in a few minutes after being carried from her chair to bed.
2. He was sent for to an obstetric case attended by a midwife; waited all day; at last a child was born in the evening. It was infra dig for so great a physician to condescend to so grovelling an act as the removal of the placenta; 'left such things to the midwife,' bade them all good night and would see patient next day. He was 'in a hurry and had an appointment'. The case being again left in the midwife's hands she tried to deliver but the 'seconds' [the placenta] would not move. After waiting a while, strong pains took place; examines and finds a head resting on the perineum! 'Bless me!' she cries, 'here's another child. Send for the doctor instantly!' The doctor was taken away, nolens volens, just as he was beginning his supper of fried salmon and strong ale (the 'appointment' to which he had been invited by a gentleman.) He was with the patient in two

hours, in time to witness the birth of a second child, dead. It is said that he, the doctor, 'looked very blue' on finding such a result of his boosted knowledge.

'In another, a forceps case, an hour or two after the delivery as he was putting on his greatcoat to leave, the women present desired him to have a look at the patient as she was snoring and puffing. He did so and found her pulseless, face exsanguine. After deluging her body and the bed with cold water he remained with her until she expired in about three hours.'

'Verax' concludes 'As such sad instances occurred rather frequently, some people expressed their surprise that any college should have made him a 'full doctor.' If we are to continue to confer the degree of MD on the illiterate and the inexperienced, it should mean 'dabbler in medicine.' If given to the grossly ignorant it should be the degree of MB, which would mean 'blunderer in medicine'.

'HEMMING, SNUFFLING, HESITATING . . . '

The *Edinburgh Monthly Journal of Medical Science* (one of the early names of *Edinburgh Medical Journal*) also believed in frank expression of opinion. This from one of its book reviews:

We have just finished the perusal of a work by Dr Gibson of Pennsylvania entitled *Rambles in Europe in 1839* in which he sketches some of the eminent physicians and surgeons of Great Britain and France. Many of these men had taught him. There is a good deal of truth and a greater quantity of impertinence displayed in some of his portraits, for example, that of Dr Home, present professor of Practice of Physic in Edinburgh and previously professor of *Materia Medica.*

Gibson writes: 'Home was never, however, distinguished as a teacher in that branch, being deficient in voice and manner. He had acquired so inherent a habit of hemming, snuffling, hesitating and recalling words as to make his lectures very unpalatable to the most of his hearers. Age, I found, had not corrected but increased these defects; and, as he never enjoyed private practice to any extent and indeed seemed to have no time for it but depended altogether for his experience on a month or two of clinical experience annually upon a few patients in the Royal Infirmary of Edinburgh, I presume his lectures on the practice of physic cannot be very edifying for his pupils. He is however a man of fine education, extensive general information, solid professional acquirements and I believe of most amiable feelings and respectable character. Though of too full habit, rather florid and beyond seventy he appears to enjoy good health and may yet live for some years.' This unflattering assessment was supported by the *Lancet*. In an editorial of 3 September 1842 they commented even more trenchantly: 'Dr Home, the Edinburgh professor of practice of physic, has been known for almost half a century as the very worst lecturer in Europe. He has at length retired and been replaced by Dr Alison. This is a judicious appointment. Alison is little given to philosophising, and to mystifying physiology by the metaphysical distinctions of the Scotch school which lead to nothing and explain nothing.'

Returning to Gibson's work he says of another man, a celebrated chemist: 'Although one for the ladies, his starchy manner, pride and formal address, led to him not being married. At the Queen's Ball he asked a lady if she was *saturated* with dancing. A rival chemist, overhearing, said: 'Hang the fellow! he ought to be *precipitated* downstairs!'

Professor James Hamilton was an obstetrician. Gibson met him when Hamilton was old but found him, in his views on some obstetrical matter, 'as opposed to Collins and other Dublin men as ever. It was both painful and amusing to see with what intellectual fire and vivacity he attacked his opponents, pulling his little red wig quickly from right to left as he spoke'.

ANOTHER POOR LECTURER

The comments on Professor Home show that poor lecturers were liable to achieve a higher profile than they might wish. Another anonymous letter, in which the victim's name is unclear, was published in the *Lancet*. The writer justifies his action by heading the letter:

> *Licuit, semperque, licebit*
> *Parcere personis, dicere de vitiis.*

a possible translation of which is: 'It has always been and it will always be permitted to allow persons to speak of vices'. He asks for action on a professor whose lectures were thought to be inadequate. He had persuaded the University Principal to attend one of the man's lectures but the result was less than had been hoped for. 'Where is the

Principal? Did he not attend *part*[*sic*] of a lecture to enforce order and attention? Did he not slip out of the lecture thereafter, quietly and with a smile on his face, leaving the professor at the mercy of the jeers of the students, well knowing the justice of their case?' He concludes 'Eloquent and talented lecturers such as Alison, Christison and Ballingall cannot make up for the inefficiency of a few of their brethren'.

SCANDAL IN THE DISSECTING ROOM

And finally 'Amicus' wrote to the *Lancet* on 12 March 1844, exposing corruption in the Edinburgh University dissecting room: 'The University has for two years now had only one demonstrator in anatomy. Because of his poor pay this man is allowed to work also as a grinder. The latter is his main concern. When in the dissecting room his attention is given exclusively to those who are engaged with him privately [i.e. those who pay him] So one must choose either to go without demonstration, or fee largely [i.e. pay generously] this double functionary.'

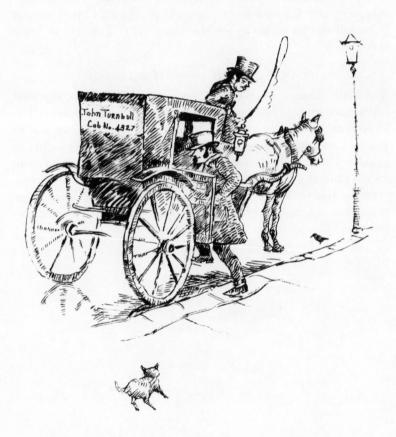

❦ 17 ❦

A very rare Disease

Sickness comes on horseback but goes away on foot.

HAZLITT

The case histories of John Turnbull and Robert Kerr are unusual. Both suffered from the same disease. Both died. No other cases of this disease are recorded in the Edinburgh pathological register for the 1840s.

JOHN TURNBULL, age unknown
Address unknown. Cab Driver.
18 November 18—. Admitted to hospital. A fortnight ago he came in from his employment complaining of a pain in his back and shivering. Thereafter he had frequently to return from work after a few hours, from languor and lassitude. He went to bed for the rest of the day but rose in the evening and drove his cab until six next morning. For a few days after this he was unable to drive but not confined to bed. He then went out for six hours but returned so much worse as to be confined to bed until admitted. During all this time he suffered severe pain in the wrists and knee joints and had a fever. The painful joints were swollen but the pustules did not appear until shortly before admission. His habits are said to have been intemperate. Had been employed in a place where it was certain that, some time ago, glandered horses had been kept.

On admission, delirious and restless but answers questions and says that he sees beasts before him. There is subsaltus tendinorum.[1] Pulse 120. There are circumscribed swellings of the wrists and of the knee joints, especially the right, not so painful as formerly, and at the same parts there is an eruption of hard circumscribed pustules or vesicles, some with an erythematous

---

[1] 'Subsaltus tendinorum' means 'tremor.'

---

border two to three lines[1] in diameter. Similar pustules also exist on the forehead. The left eye is completely closed by a swelling of the upper lid and corresponding side of the nose. On the trunk and extremities pustules are also here presenting the same characteristics. There is considerable cough with râles at the front of the chest. Breathing rapid and distressed. Subsequent to admission he fell into a deep sleep accompanied by profuse perspiration.

Vespere: Applic: emplastrum vesic: 6 x 4 sterno.[2]

℞ *Extr: Aloes* grains 12. *Calomelanos* grains 12. *Opii* grains 4. *Cons: Rosanum q l.. ut fiat pil. 8 sumat 1 sexta qq hora.*[3] *Hab: Vin: Rubr: 3 ounces.*[4]

19 November 18—. Bowels open this morning. Perspiring profusely. Dyspnoea.

℞ Carb: Ammon: 1 drachm. Aqua Fontis 3 oz. Aqua Cinnamonii 3 oz. *Sumat ½ oz.* [illegible][5] *Hab: Vin Rubr:* 8 ounces

Vespere. ℞ *Sulph: Quinae* 3 grains. *Pulv: Aromat:* 3 grains. *Fiat Pulv. Sumat 1 hora somni et repetua cras mané*[6]

[1] A 'line' is an old unit of measurement equivalent to one-twelfth of an inch.

[3] 'A blistering agent to be applied, as a plaster six inches by four inches, to the sternum.'

[4] Calomelanos (calomel or subchloride of mercury) was a preparation of mercury popular in Edinburgh. Beasley states that it has many uses, and 'as its operation is uncertain it is usual to combine it with a vegetable purgative' (here aloes). The rose preparation was simply a vehicle, the amount here being '*q l* or '*quantum lubet* which means 'as much as you please.' Eight pills were to be made and one given every six hours.

[5] 'To have 3 oz. of red wine'. Red wine was often given to the very seriously ill.

[5] This mixture of ammonium carbonate, aqua fontis ('spring water') and cinnamon was probably given with the intention of increasing diaphoresis. (A further and dramatic use of ammonia – here the caustic liqor ammoniae – is quoted by Beasley. Napoleon Bonaparte required treatment 'for the immediate cure of severe hoarseness'. A Dr Foreau prescribed ten drops of liqor ammoniae to be mixed with one and a half ounces of syrup of erysimum (the crucifer known as hedge mustard) and three ounces of the infusion of tilia, an infusion derived from the lime tree. The mixture was to be taken as a single dose. The result of treatment is not recorded.)

[6] Quinine was given for fever. Pulvis aromaticus was the Edinburgh name for compound powder of cinnamon. It contained cinnamon, cardamom and ginger. One dose was to be given 'at the hour of sleep', the other the following morning.

He continued in the same condition till 2 am when he began to sink rapidly and died at 4 am.

Diagnosis in ward journal – glanders.

Sectio cadaveris

[extracts taken from the Edinburgh pathological register]

In addition to the external appearances a pustule similar to those on the skin was found above the right chorda vocalis and similar smaller ones on the mucous surface of the trachea. Mucopurulent material in bronchi. The lungs had scattered ecchymosed subpleural patches.

On opening the nasal cavities [only done because the disease was suspected in life] a line of small circular excavations was observed to extend along the line between the inferior and middle turbinate bones which was infiltrated with pus, the opposite side being free from ulceration.

Examination otherwise normal.

Summary of findings 'Glanders. Recent pustules skin and integument, epiglottis, larynx, trachea and lungs. Pus between frontal bone and dura mater. Old lesions lungs and mesenteric glands. ? old syphilis.' (signed W. T. Gairdner)

ROBERT KERR, aged 61

Address unknown. Omnibus Driver

Turnbull was a cab driver; Robert Kerr drove an omnibus. Craigie published an account of Kerr's case in the *Edinburgh Medical and Surgical Journal* (Vol. 59, 1843, p. 123). The title of the paper was 'A case in which the symptoms of Acute Farcy appeared in the human subject'.

Craigie 'thought it important to publish', as it was 'the first case as far as is known in which the disease was recognised in life in Scotland.' He goes on 'when the eruption appeared, the idea presented itself to me that it was similar to Farcy and had there been a discharge from the nose I would have called it Glanders. This was confirmed by a friend who had seen a case of Glanders in London. Kerr closely resembled that one, apart from absence of nasal discharge. I had never seen one, all my knowledge being from papers of Dr Elliotson and M. Rayer. Kerr groomed his own horses and three weeks before admission there had been two horses with glanders in the stables where his horses were kept. It was not possible to confirm actual contact. At post-mortem Kerr's nostrils were normal, as far as dissected."

The ward Journal in which this man's history and progress were written is no longer in existence. Luckily the pathologist copied the clinical record into the Edinburgh Pathological Register as a preliminary to writing up the post-mortem findings. It is as follows:

11 November 1841. Admitted to Dr Craigie's care. He was in a state of delirium and unable to give an account of himself. He was stated to have been ill for eight days, with delirium, pain of head, diarrhoea and occasional vomiting.

On examination the delirium was of the low muttering kind. The hands and lower jaw were affected with a constant tremor. Constant motion of subsaltus tendinorum. Pulse small and rapid. Marks of old ulcers were found on lips and recent impetiginous-looking scabs mixed with blotches of a dull red colour, in some places swelling and beginning to suppurate. On the chin was a large scabbed blister of similar description.

17 November 1841. Passed a good night and more intelligent today. The trembling of the lips and the *subsaltus tendinorum* however continue and he can only imperfectly protrude the tongue.

18 November 1841. Pulse 112, respirations 44. Imperfect consciousness. On left side of chin there is a diffuse red swelling, closely set with small white pustules of which some discharge bloody serum.

19 November 1841. Became more collapsed. The pustules on the chin coalescing. On lower extremities are numerous vesicles surrounded by a red areola at the base with an elevated round summit containing white opaque matter. The larger pustules referred to on admission have no suppuration but now include the whole thickness of the integument although they show no tendency to point or burst. He remained partially conscious until his death at 6 pm. The blisters had increased in size.'

Before describing the post-mortem findings the pathologist added 'This case was but little understood during life and the post-mortem did not in the least solve the mystery that hung about it. On enquiry after death it appeared that, though the horses he was driving were healthy, they were near now glanderous horses in the stables belonging to the same party for whom he worked, but in which his horses were not kept [*sic*]. Seemed probable that he might have received some glanderous material into his constitution. The symptoms he laboured under very closely resembled those described as constituting the 'acute farcy glanders.' He had throughout no running from the nostrils either before admission or while in hospital.

Sectio cadaveris

A stout man the whole body studded with pustules containing a thick opaque white pus, interspersed in places with smaller or larger subcutaneous abscesses which showed no ulceration but rather a tendency to spread in the cellular tissue, the integument covering them being of a livid hue. Legs covered in similar spots with scars of old ulcers.

The brain displays a copious subarachnoid effusion by which the membranes at the posterior part of the hemisphere are elevated above the level of the convolutions. The ventricles contain fully two ounces of very clear serum and a considerable amount was also found at the base.

In the right lung is a large gangrenous abscess not distinctly circumscribed but surrounded by lung tissue condensed by influx of partially [illegible], infiltrated with pus. Lower lobes fully crepitant. Left lung shows recent inflammation.

Purulent deposits were found on the surface of the frontal and parietal bones and in the deep-seated tissues of the neck. [Craigie's paper adds that 'the nostrils were normal as far as dissected'.]'

NOTES ON GLANDERS

1. Glanders is a contagious disease of horses, other equids and some cats, which can affect man. The cause is pseudomonas mallei. It is one of the oldest diseases known and at one time was worldwide The contact between horses in time of war increased its spread. The French, for example, slaughtered twenty thousand horses in the Great War. In the second World War the German army had five thousand cases in south- east Europe alone.

The pathology in humans is that of a chronic granuloma leading to a purulent infection of mucous membranes which may end in necrosis of cartilage and bone. There may be an eruption of skin nodules and there is a septicaemic form of which Kerr's case is a particularly good example. The illness has also been called 'malleus', and there is a more chronic form called 'farcy'. These terms vary with different authors. Farcy was suspected by Craigie in Kerr's case, where the full clinical notes are missing.

2. In 1995 the British Ministry of Agriculture warned in what is still the most up-to-date issue of its 'Exotic Disease Series' [No. 6 pp.17–20], 'glanders has been eradicated from Europe, North America and Oceania. Currently it exists in the Middle East, India, Pakistan and some other Asiatic and African countries with low sporadic incidence. In Myanmar (Burma), Mongolia and China the disease appears to be widespread.' Border controls on imported equids have to be strictly applied in countries where the disease has been eradicated. In 1998, for example, it is believed, though it has not been confirmed, that France found a seropositive horse on checking animals imported from Rumania.

3. In the *Bulletin du L'Academie Royale de Medicin* of 7 February 1843, quoted in the *Edinburgh Medical and Surgical Journal* [Vol. LX, 1843, p. 263], A. M. Renault describes how he injected a horse with pus taken from a man with glanders. 'The horse was soon thereafter seized with the disease. Before killing it, 10 mls. of its jugular blood was injected into a healthy horse. This also developed glanders, after three days. The procedure was repeated into another horse, with the same result in three days.' Renault's conclusion was 'The blood is essentially diseased in this fearful malady.'

4. The early editions of the *Book of the Horse* by S. Sidney published by Cassell, Petter and Galpin, appeared more than one hundred years ago. They contain the following entry: 'This fatal, infectious and mysterious disease exposes the owner of an infected horse to such severe penalties that if the animal is of small value and the suspicion strong, the better plan is to kill it and burn the body in a lime kiln if it cannot be buried too deep for dogs to get at it in the earth. The earliest symptom is a discharge from the nostril, small in quantity, *constantly flowing* [*sic*]. It flows from one nostril, generally the left or offside one [*sic*]. The horse may be at the time in perfect working condition. It should at once be separated from its companions and

medical advice sought.' A public notice issued by London County Council in 1892 confirmed that people were aware of the danger. It required that any case of glanders or farcy be notified to the police. Failure to notify meant a fine of £20.

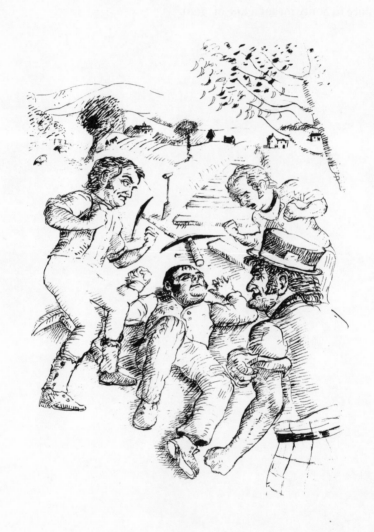

❦ 18 ❦

The Infirmary and the Railways

I've been workin' on the railroad
All the live-long day.

American Popular Song

As the decade of the 1840s went on, 'the race for the Border' intensified. Anderson, in his History of Edinburgh, reports rivalry among railway companies to be the first to link Scotland and England. In 1846 the North British Railway Company opened its line from Edinburgh to North Berwick. On 9 April 1847 the foundation stone of Edinburgh's Caledonian Station was laid and in 1848 the Caledonian Railway opened its line to Carlisle going via Currie and Beattock.

Light railways had been used earlier, in a small way, to carry the coal previously moved by canal. The first proper passenger railway to operate wholly within Scotland was the service between Edinburgh and Glasgow which 'cut the journey from four hours to two.' The opening ceremony of that line was reported by Anderson as follows:

'On 18 February 1842 a train of thirty carriages arrived at mid-day from Glasgow, drawn by the three engines *Stevenson, Playfair* and *Galileo.* The band of the 53rd Regiment welcomed the train, playing 'See, the conquering hero comes!' The Edinburgh directors of the company then entered their train, of twenty-six carriages, and both trains left for Glasgow travelling at 15–25 miles per hour.'

Work on the other railways continued, providing regular work over several years for large numbers of labourers. The workmen were both local men and Irishmen driven out of their country by the potato famine. On 17 November 1845 a letter was sent from the Infirmary board to the North British Railway Company. This called the company's attention to the number of accidents and other cases involving people in their employment, and solicited a subscription to the funds of the hospital. The Edinburgh Royal Infirmary, it pointed out, had been built to serve the people of Edinburgh and district and it depended on the generosity of local people for its funding. The many Irishmen now in the area had placed an extra financial burden on the hospital and it seemed fair that the employers be asked to help.

To begin with the response was slow. The board's minutes show a donation of £5 5s. from the Edinburgh and Glasgow Railway Company in 1846. On 22 March 1847 Dr Christison got the Infirmary board to write again to the North British Railway Company's directors about the number of patients being admitted from Middleton Muir, one of the railway construction camps. For one reason or another there were ninety-three railway labourers in the Infirmary on one day in the early part of that year. The board wished the three railway companies, the North British, the Caledonian, and the Edinburgh and Northern to pay the cost of their employees' admissions. This time all the companies paid up, the Edinburgh and North. making 'a very satisfactory and liberal donation'.

The men whose case notes are reproduced here were all railway workers.

DAVID BRENNAN, aged 25
Canonmills. Initially Belfast. A labourer.
24 May 1841. Admitted to surgical wards of Professor Syme having sustained a comminuted fracture a little below the middle of the right femur from a fall of earth on the new line of railway between Edinburgh and Newhaven. There is considerable swelling with two inches of shortening and eversion of the foot.

The limb was extended and a pasteboard splint placed on each side of the thigh and Desault's long splint applied.
2 July 1841. Splint removed. Limb of proper length and firmly united. Two pasteboard splints applied with a bandage.
August. Limb firmly united and of proper length. Had strabismus of the left eye for which the internal rectus was divided about ten days ago with perfect success, both eyes being quite straight after the operation. No bad effects followed it.
Date unknown. Dismissed cured.

PATRICK MCPHIE, aged 35
From County Monaghan. A labourer on the railway.
13 May 1841. Admitted to surgical wards of Professor Syme, on account of bruising of the left side of the chest sustained by having been knocked down by a fall of earth while working on the Glasgow Railway three days ago. Before admission he had suffered severe pain on drawing his breath for which he had been twice freely bled from his arm with great relief. There is now no swelling and no fracture can be detected.

Rest and a flannel roller.
17 May 1841. Dismissed cured. R.M.

MICHAEL SINCLAIR, aged 32
Kirkliston. A labourer.
29 June 1841. Admitted to surgical wards of Professor Syme. Yesterday, while working on the railway, was assaulted by a number of men and knocked down by a blow on the head from a pick shaft. While trying to defend himself he was repeatedly struck over the hands and different parts of the body.

On examination there is great swelling of both hands and crepitus over the two first metacarpal heads of the right hand. Two suppurating puncture wounds are found on the crown of the head, in the higher of which the bone is exposed.

Poultices applied to the head and fomentations to the hands.
10 July 1841. Dismissed cured.

IAN CROMBIE, aged 51
Easter Duddingston. A railway labourer.
5 June 1849. Admitted to hospital. The following statement is from friends, his own memory having failed.

Eight or nine years since, he was of intemperate habits but four or five years ago he entirely relinquished the use of intoxicating liquors. About two or three years ago he began to complain of loss of eyesight and swelling of the face. This continued till nine months ago when, besides these symptoms, he became weak in the intellect. He was then, according to reports, eating turnips with sugar spread on them under the impression that it was buttered bread, and going out with his clothes turned outside in. He never, however, became in any way outrageous in his conduct. His friends attributed his mental change to working with naphthalene. He was attended at that time by Dr Hill, Portobello, and in two months he was so far recovered as to resume work as a plate layer on the North British Railway. He continued at this until five months ago when he was again seized with the same complaint but with more swelling of the face and limbs and of the abdomen which was so distended as to prevent his clothes from going on. This state of matters continued until eleven days ago when, as he was stooping to pick up something, he became apparently stiff and fell upon the floor in a bent posture with rigidity of the muscles of the legs and complete loss of sensibility This fit was repeated the next day and these were the only two he ever had. He has remained in much the same way until admitted.

On examination some headache, no giddiness. Sight impaired and squints with right eye. He did not do so some months before. Pupils do not contract to usual size upon stimulus with light. No pain except in head. Some oedema of face and abdomen. No loss of power or feeling in any part. Pulse 60, intensity at times outwith heart sounds' natural.

℞ *Pulv: Jalap Co:* 1 drachm [*sic*].[1] *App: Cuc.*[2]

6 June 1849. Head easier since cupping last night. Says his recollection is more distinct.

18 June 1849. Dismissed cured.

Diagnosis in ward journal – head affection.

---

[1] As always, purgation was felt to be necessary

[2] 'App: Cuc:' means 'apply cucurbitula' i.e. 'apply cupping glass'.

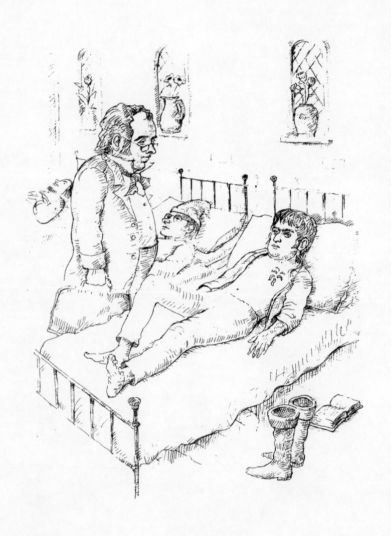

❦ 19 ❦

Cupping, Leeching and other Activities

My times be in thy hand!
Perfect the cup as planned!
ROBERT BROWNING, *Rabbi Ben Ezra*

Much of the oral medication administered in hospitals in the 1840s was unpleasant, both in taste and in its effects. Many of the substances used were ineffective and some were dangerous. In addition, uncomfortable physical treatments were used, which were at times just as dangerous. It is not surprising, therefore, that many patients reported themselves to be remarkably better, remarkably quickly! It is also no surprise to find many case records marked, 'absconded' or 'left hospital irregularly'. Mrs Murray from the Pleasance, for example, reported herself 'considerably relieved' after one treatment. The day before, four leeches had been applied around her anus for 'great irritability of the uterus'.

The commoner physical treatments were cupping, leeching, venesection, acupuncture, galvanism, the cautery, cataplasms, blistering, shaving the head and the use of setons. Often more than one procedure was employed. Three involved blood letting and in two of these it was the considered necessary to remove the blood as near to the perceived site of the problem as possible. The treatments are briefly discussed here, with case histories which illustrate the indications for which they were prescribed.

CUPPING

This method of withdrawal of blood involved the use of a 'cupping glass' with scarification of the skin. The cup was first warmed and then pressed to the skin which had, at that place been scarified. As the glass cooled a partial vacuum formed within it, this and the scarification increasing the blood flow. '*Cucurbitula cruentā*' meant 'a cupping glass with scarificator'. The prescriber indicated the site and Mr Cope the cupper, or a deputy, arrived to carry out the procedure. In 1841 it was pointed out by the junior Infirmary doctors that Mr Cope, who had started work at the Infirmary in 1831 had never received payment, either for his work or for the expense of providing cupping glasses and instruments. In addition he had recently been the sole cupper. The board put this right and by January 1846 his pay had gone up to £21 per annum. On one occasion, a cupper-whether Mr Cope or not is not stated-refused to cup a fever case. He was told he would be sacked if this was repeated.

COLIN PATERSON, aged 34
Grassmarket. A slater
31 May 1841. Admitted to the surgical wards of Professor Syme. A few hours before admission, while cleaning a window, he overbalanced himself and fell backwards to the ground, a distance of fifteen feet, pitching on the back of his shoulder. He rose immediately and walked a short way but soon afterwards became nearly insensible and was unable to move his lower extremities.

On examination can move limbs freely and has no complaint but of pain and stiffness in the lower part of the dorsal region of his spine. The spine of the 10th dorsal vertebra is found prominent and a distinct depression exists between it and the spine of the ninth. A good deal of swelling around the parts with tenderness over the projecting spine.

Fomentations were applied. Two cupping glasses applied in the evening and twelve ounces of blood withdrawn.
1 June 1841. Less swelling and tenderness.
3 June 1841. Pain on motion; a flannel roller applied.
15 June 1841. Less pain on motion
10 July 1841. Gaining strength. Now walks about the greater part of the day. Still complains of weakness of back.
18 July 1841. Dismissed cured.

LEECHES

In the wild these are ectoparasites on vertebrates. They attach themselves firmly to a passing host and then draw blood, for which purpose they were used in hospital. They could also be bought independently in Edinburgh for home use. Those supplied to the Infirmary came from L. Friedlander, the board's accounts for the quarter ended 31 December 1844 including the item: 'Friedlander, L. Leeches £23 18s. 4d.'

The Infirmary apothecary arranged with the board for the appointment of one woman 'to have the entire charge of applying leeches to the patients and of looking after the leeches when removed. She could also be of use otherwise in the House.' The apothecary compared figures for the numbers of leeches used between 1 February and 31 July in 1839 and in 1840. The minutes note that 'the saving of about half the number afforded the managers much satisfaction'.

MAGNUS CUMMING, aged 45
Shetland. A fisherman.
21 December 1849. Admitted to surgical wards of Professor Syme. Fifteen months ago fell eight feet in the hold of a vessel on to left shoulder. Felt sharp pain on left side of chest which was limited to a very small part and resembled the pain of a knife striking him. He was relieved with a little rum and water but since then the pain is pretty constant, going down left arm and causing tingling of left fingers. On examination no abnormal signs of any kind.
22 December 1849. Apply leeches 6 *regioni cordis.*[1]
23 December 1849. Leeches bled freely.
24 December 1849. He had an attack of epistaxis last night and the pain is now much diminished.
5 January 1850. A blister and three more leeches have been applied and he now feels really well.
7 January 1850. Dimissed cured.

[1] 'Apply six leeches to the region of the heart.'

VENESECTION

The third and most efficient method of removal of blood was by venesection. The amount to be removed was indicated by the doctor in charge of the patient and the procedure carried out by the clerk. If the amount was not specified, the aim was to continue bleeding until the patient showed signs of imminent syncope.

A remarkable example of the use of this form of treatment is recounted in the case of David Brown at the end of this book.

ACUPUNCTURE

This was carried out in time-honoured fashion.

HENRY MORRISON, aged 30

Dunfermline. A weaver.

6 June 1844. Admitted to Professor Syme's wards. Three months ago, when recovering from smallpox, he was exposed to cold and wet. He has since complained of pain shooting from the hip along the posterior aspect of the thigh and passing behind and to the outer side of the knee whence it shoots down both the anterior and posterior aspects of the leg and along the sole of the foot. The course of the pain corresponds to the position and distribution of the great sciatic nerve.

7 June 1844. Acupuncture needles have been today inserted along the course of the sciatic nerve at those spots where the pain was most acute, two in the region of the hip, one at the ankle.

8 June 1844. The pain is today considerably relieved.

23 June 1844. Discharged relieved.   Kelburne King

GALVANISM

Galvanism meant the application of direct electrical current produced by chemical action in a battery. Named after Luigi Galvani (1737–98). The electrodes were applied to the skin wrapped in sponges.

ALASTAIR BLACK, aged 29

Canongate. A flesher.

9 June 1845. Admitted. States he was in Dr Paterson's ward about fifteen months ago with dyspepsia and a very large discharge of urine amounting sometimes, as he says, to 'forty pounds a day'. He is not aware that it was ever sweet. The books cannot be found to authenticate this statement. [Nor can they today.]

30 June 1845. Feels still very weak and desponding but no vomiting. Ordered to be weighed and to have galvanism transmitted through the region of his stomach.

1 July 1845. Galvanism applied last night for a quarter of an hour.

Says he feels better today and has more appetite.

2 July 1845. The Galvanism to be applied again this evening.

5 July 1845. He says he is tired of living in a hospital and wishes to be dismissed that he may try the effects of some more outdoor exercise. Dismissed – no change.

Diagnosis in ward register – diabetes insipidus.

THE CAUTERY

There were two types of cautery. The 'actual cautery' or white-hot iron, and the 'potential cautery', a caustic substance. While some considered the actual cautery barbaric, A. T. Thomson, in his *Elements of Materia Medica and Therapeutics* written in 1835, confirms that the iron was indeed applied directly to the skin at the appropriate site. Thomson gives clear directions on how it should be done. It is possible that, in some cases, some protection was used to diffuse the heat.

KATE McCUISH, aged 22

Dundee. Factory girl (a reeler).

3 July 1844. Admitted to surgical wards of Professor Syme having, about three months ago, struck her left shoulder with a basket of lint. It immediately became painful and she lost the use of her left arm to a considerable extent. A week later she applied to a bone-setter who, stating that the arm was out of joint, made several attempts to reduce the so-called dislocation. The pain steadily increased and the arm became gradually weaker.

On admission she complains of severe pain in the shoulder extending down the arm which is felt more at night. The deltoid is atrophied and the arm retains but little power of motion.

8 July 1844. The actual cautery was today applied anteriorly and behind the shoulder joint.

9 July 1844. Since the application of the cautery she has not felt any of the deep-seated pain of which she originally complained.

12 September [*sic*] She can now raise her hand to her head. Dismissed cured.   Kelburne King

---

CATAPLASMS

These were also known as 'poultices' or 'plasters' and were used for local heating or for counter-irritation. The *British Pharmacopoeia* of 1867 listed six varieties: charcoal, hemlock, yeast, linseed, mustard and chlorine [*sic*]. The last involved mixing 'linseed meal with boiling water and slowly adding a solution of chlorinated soda with constant stirring'. One unfortunate, Graham Morton, found himself in hospital in July 1844 after someone had tried, a year before, to cure a hard lump on his nose with a plaster of corrosive sublimate. This had produced an ulcer 'which has never since shown any disposition to heal'. The efforts of Professor Syme were equally unsuccessful, his clerk, Kelburne King, noting that 'the ulcer is stationary. He wishes to go home and is accordingly dismissed'. Marion McPhail's story is more orthodox.

MARION McPHAIL, aged 23
Edinburgh. A servant.
24 November 1845. Admitted to ward? Thinks she caught cold on the 11th after being exposed to wet. On the 17th and subsequent days she felt rather unwell and had some pain in the loins. Became feverish on the evening of the 20th with back pain and headache which continued till the evening of Sunday the 23rd when a papular eruption appeared on the arm and hands. After its appearance the symptoms abated in severity. Had a slight bronchial affection for which a large cataplasm has been applied to the chest the evening before admission. [She went on to develop a vesicular eruption, probably smallpox modified by vaccination, from which she recovered]

BLISTERING

Cantharides, a preparation made from 'Spanish fly' (a beetle, lytta vesicatoria) was described by Beasley as 'the most usual and convenient basis of blistering compounds'. It was used either as a liquid, a liniment or as a blistering paper. The latter was often ruled in one-inch squares. This enabled the prescriber to indicate clearly the size of the area to be blistered.

JOHN HUME, aged 43
Greenock. A canvas weaver
7 May 1841. Admitted to the surgical wards of Professor Syme.
About twelve months ago, and with no assignable reason, he felt
a darting pain to pass through his right hand near its root. This
continued for fourteen weeks and occasionally extended as high
as the elbow. More severe at night and in damp weather. He has
employed mustard and fly blisters, various liniments, warm bath-
ing. Under the use of them the pain has somewhat diminished.
 There is now fullness of the anterior part of the root of the
hand and wrist with distinct synovial crepitus and fluctuation.
℞ A blister to be applied along the seat of the fullness and pain.
8 May 1841. Blister rose well. To have a catharctic draught.
14 May 1841. The fluid has been made to bulge in the palm of the
hand. Two drachms of thin glairy fluid were evacuated, containing
small flat bodies like fish scales. Bandaged.
24 May 1841. Dismissed with advice.   Richard McKenzie

SHAVING THE HEAD

This was a common practice in head injuries and in medical conditions associated with loss of consciousness from any cause. Terence
Booth was admitted in July 1845, unconscious and with a hemiplegia.
Various treatments were used without improvement and finally the
instruction was given to *abradat: capilli et admot: hirudines X dextra
lateri capitis* (i.e. shave the hair of the head and apply ten leeches to the
right side of the head). He died.

SETONS

Setons were drains. They consisted of a skein of silk introduced by a
special needle at the relevant site. A fold of skin was pinched-up, the
needle carrying the silk pushed through and the needle detached. The
silk was thought to allow drainage and the hole was kept open by an
oily preparation. In addition to drainage of purulent material, setons
were also considered useful in some cases of apoplexy and palsy. Jemima
Angus, whose case is summarised below, had one inserted in her neck.

COMBINATIONS OF THE ABOVE TREATMENTS

(partly summarised)

THOMAS SMITH, aged 25
9 Greenside Place. Chimney Sweep.
Admitted unconscious with a diagnosis of apoplexy and delirium tremens. He made a complete recovery. During his admission his head was shaved. Cold cloths were applied to head. Twelve leeches were applied to the temples. A drop of croton oil was placed on tongue with sugar and was to be repeated in an hour if necessary. A strait-jacket was applied. He was given a turpentine enema and an ice-bag was placed on his head. Whisky and a morphine draught were given at night.

HELEN ADAMSON, aged 26
Canongate. A servant.
While cleaning a room, suddenly raised her head and struck it forcibly against the edge of a table. She complained of headache thereafter. In hospital she was given various medicines and had the posterior part of her head shaved and twelve leeches applied behind the left ear. Acupuncture needles were inserted. As there was no improvement Mr Syme was invited to see her in the medical ward. He ordered a blister over the left parietal bone and tablets of ferrous carbonate.

JEMIMA ANGUS, aged 26
140 Cowgate. Husband a baker.
Admission date unknown. In November last when, while washing the floor, a large soup plate fell from between four and five feet above her and broke upon her head. She was stunned but not unconscious. Well in two days. In March she had a sudden severe headache in front of coronal suture, the site of the November injury. Since the first appearance of headache her sight has always been liable to be affected. She has now lost nearly the whole use of the left eye the pupil of which seems permanently contracted.

She applied for relief at the New Town dispensary where her head was shaved, blistered and rubbed with croton oil. Six leeches were applied to the fore part of head. She was blistered and cupped at the back of the neck. All with little relief. She was then admitted here to ward 13 but discharged in four days without any

treatment as 'improper' on account of supposed mania. She returned here and a seton was introduced at the back of the neck on
Friday last. This is now discharging but not freely. Eight leeches
applied. She was dismissed relieved.

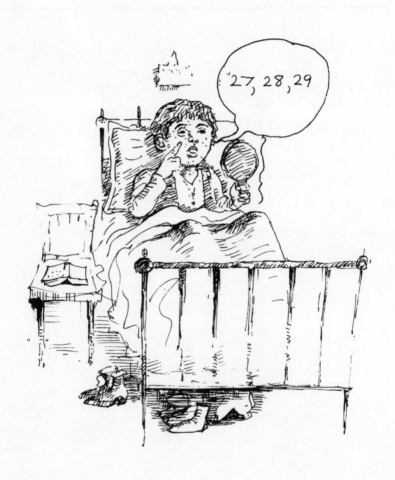

❦ 20 ❦

Smallpox and Measles

That dire disease, whose ruthless power
Withers the beauty's transient flower
GOLDSMITH, *The Double Transformation*

Smallpox was not uncommon in Edinburgh in the mid-nineteenth century. Edward Jenner of Gloucestershire had described smallpox vaccination as far back as 1798. Edinburgh citizens now had the option of being vaccinated by choice although there was as yet no formal public vaccination programme in the city. The disease was more dreaded than measles although the latter was often fatal.

SMALLPOX

While a smallpox patient might still be admitted to an ordinary medical ward, there was a growing awareness of the need for isolation. Ward 8 in the Royal was set aside for smallpox cases in March 1840. In November 1842 there was another peak in the number of cases which led to Mrs Wood, the matron requesting that the managers 'open the room at the top of the stairs for female smallpox patients'.

The disease was not always fatal but, as Macaulay said, 'it leaves on those whose lives it spares, the hideous traces of its power'. One man, a canal worker, was admitted with an unrelated illness. The clerk who wrote him up described him as being 'of florid complexion, robust and strongly marked with the smallpox'.

The cases of Constance Brown and Marion Hynd are typical of many others. The stories of Cathy Johnston and her infant son Leonard are more unusual.

CONSTANCE BROWN, aged 13
Child of pensioner
10 March 1849. Admitted to ward 11. States that on the 4th, six days ago, had shivering in the morning and felt cold all day with great heats. Had great headache, much thirst and complete loss of appetite. During the next two days, the same symptoms and, in addition, great weakness of back and some vomiting.

On the morning of the fourth day (7th inst.) the surface of the body was covered with a red rash and the face and shoulders were studded with numerous small pimples. She had much sweating. Next day the pimples appeared in other parts. Since then has continued much the same. Has had no food, no sleep, much thirst and frequent vomiting.

On admission complains of sore throat and slight cough. There is much uneasiness from the state of the surface. The face, arms, and back are covered with a copious eruption of rounded, flattened, whitish umbilicated vesicles. These are somewhat confluent on face around the mouth and nose and on the cheeks. There are one or two confluent patches on the arms.

The eruption is much less copious on the lower limbs and anterior surface of trunk where the vesicles are redder and less advanced. The eyelids are considerably swollen and vesicles are seen on their margins. The conjunctivae are red and somewhat oedematous. The tongue is pretty thickly studded with vesicles. Deglutition painful. Pulse 90, rather small.

There is a distinct vaccine mark on the upper part of the left arm. Her father states that she was vaccinated. The day before she was taken ill she had been in a house where there was a child ill of smallpox. [Too recent to be the source of infection but perhaps she had visited that child earlier]

12 March 1849. Eruption very confluent on face and arms, vesicles with depressed centres and full of fluid. Some tendency to encrustation on the face. Some swelling of the face. Tongue presents numerous vesicles. Pulse 100.

19 March 1849. Slowly improving since maturation completed. Fever gone. To have steak diet.

28 March 1849. Is still improving.

7 May 1849. Discharged cured.

MARION HYND, aged 6
Address not known
5 June 1849. Admitted ward 11. An account of her condition previous to admission has not been obtained but she was said to have been ill for ten days.

The face, body and limbs are covered with an eruption of vesicles surrounded by red bases with depressed apices and containing opaque fluid. Some of those on the face are coherent and partially encrusted. No vaccine marks to be observed. Skin warm. Throat swollen and red and there is some cough.

[During her admission she was treated with Dover's powder,[1] various purgatives and red wine]

6 June 1849. Has slept after powder. Hoarse cough continues.
9 June 1849. Encrustation is going on without itching. Pulse nearly natural.
21 June 1849. Has gradually got quite well and is now going about the ward.
14 June 1849. Dismissed cured.
Diagnosis in ward register – *Variola sine vacc.*[2]

CATHY JOHNSTON, aged 22
and her infant son LEONARD BLACK, aged 10 months
Address not known.
4 December 1844. Admitted to medical ward. States that she enjoyed good health until the first of this month when she was troubled with pain and swelling in the lips and in the right cheek. Has often been troubled with toothache and has many decayed teeth in her gums at present.

On examination appears stout and healthy. The right cheek is considerably swollen so that she can with difficulty open the jaw on this side. There is much heat and redness in the part. From the symptoms she appears to be labouring under erysipelas. An active

---

[1] Dover's powder consisted of 'ipecacuanha, opium and sulphate of potash'. This was Beasley's recipe. He describes it as 'one of the most useful sudorifics we possess. Used in febrile states and 'is a good means of giving opiates in small quantities to children'.

[2] 'Smallpox without vaccination.'

purge was administered accompanied with warm fomentations to the cheek.

5 December 1844. The swelling and pain have rather abated and the redness diminished. Dr Dunsmore opened an abscess which had formed on the inside of the cheek with much relief. A poultice was then ordered to the cheek and a strong purging mixture given.

7 December 1844. Much better. The swelling has greatly subsided and she complains of little pain. The child is suffering from eczema impetiginoides on the scalp for which no treatment is thought necessary.

17 December 1844. The infant now has as a papular eruption on the face, body and extremities. It was perceived to be unwell since the 14th, coughing and refusing its food but not so urgent as to require any treatment until this morning when the eruption was first perceived. It was ordered to have a warm bath.

18 December 1844. From the existence of a severe case of smallpox in the ward it was thought right to vaccinate the child today.

20 December 1844. The whole surface is covered with vesicles which, however, are not so numerous as to become confluent. They are more numerous on the face.

22 December 1844. The characteristic pustules of smallpox are now fully apparent all over the infant's body. In a few parts of the face they are becoming confluent. The face was ordered to be kept constantly covered with oil or lard. It is much swollen as are the extremities.

29 December 1844. The pustules having become rough and being broken, numerous small crusts are seen, of a dark colour.

30 December 1844. The child is suffering this morning from acute bronchitis from exposure to cold. This is in consequence of its mother constantly undressing it to examine the eruption. An abscess about the size of a shilling is to be found on the back on the last dorsal vertebra. It was ordered to be poulticed.

2 January 1845. The child has almost ceased coughing. Many of the scabs are falling off leaving cicatrices. The boil on the back was opened yesterday from which a small slough has come out. To continue the poultice.

5 January 1845. Nitrate of silver was applied to the boil today as it was not looking healthy.

---

11 January 1845. The ulcer is looking healthy. The water dressing ordered to be applied. The crusts on the face and body have fallen off leaving depressions.

Today the mother was ordered discharged for misbehaviour and consequently the child is discharged also.

C.H. [Charles Harwood]

MEASLES

'Did you have the measles', asked Artemus Ward, an American, 'and if so how many?' Strangely this was written in the nineteenth century when the disease, being often fatal, was somewhat less than amusing! The Christie family would not have laughed too loudly. After the Christies, Patricia Muir and her two relatives present a different problem, namely the difficulty of distinguishing between measles, typhoid and typhus in the early stages.

PATRICK CHRISTIE, aged 9
Address unknown
12 April 1847. Admitted to hospital. Four days before admission was seized with a rigor, headache and slight nausea. Also some cough. One of his brothers died a day or two ago from measles.

On examination complains of headache and thirst. Coughs and sneezes a great deal. A slight measly eruption is visible on chest and abdomen.
8 May 1847. Dismissed cured.

FRANK CHRISTIE, aged 6
Address unknown
24 April 1847. Admitted to hospital. This boy is a second brother of Patrick Christie and is also affected with measles.
8 May 1847. Dismissed cured.

PATRICIA MUIR, aged 25
High Street, Edinburgh. A housewife.
23 January 1846. Admitted to hospital. Was taken ill on the 18th with rigors, pain in the head and other symptoms of fever. The chilliness and rigors remained until after admission. This morning the headache is better. The skin is hot but perspirable. Had

---

considerable sense of heat through the night. Bowels not moved since admission. Pulse 120. Doubtful eruption of rose-coloured spots.

24 January 1846. Measles eruption now most marked on face, body and arms.

25 January 1846. Is not aware of any exposure to infection, except assisting to chest[1] her sister who died of fever on 1st January.

26 January 1846. Eruption faded. Skin cool.

10 February 1846. Dismissed cured.[2]

MARY GILLESPIE, aged 5
(The niece of Patricia Muir)
23 January 1846. Admitted to hospital. Was taken ill on the 21st in the morning, refusing her food and complaining of pain in the belly. Less so on admission. Pulse 135.

24 January 1846. This morning is marked with the typhoid eruption (4th day). Her mother died of fever on the New Year's Day [*sic*] and she has lived since with her aunt, the preceding case in this ward journal [i.e. Patricia Muir].

26 January 1846. Eruption still distinct on some parts. Pulse 120.

10 February 1846. Dismissed cured.

[1] 'To chest' is to put in a coffin.

[2] It looks as if the diagnosis in these three patients was the same but it is difficult to be sure if it was typhoid, typhus or measles. The incubation period in Patricia Muir's case suggests that, if she caught it from her sister, measles is probably the least likely although this very speculative.

UNUSUAL CASES FROM THE JOURNALS: IV

SEAN CROPPER, aged 17
From Night Asylum. A labourer on the tramp.
11 August 1842. Admitted to hospital. States that five days ago, when on his way here from Glasgow, he was seized with severe rigors, general pain and anorexia. He continued his journey for two days till he reached Edinburgh, the rigors repeatedly recurring. Since then he has been at the night asylum.[1]
On examination face flushed, skin hot. Is intelligent but answers questions slowly. Eyes slightly bloodshot. Pulse 110.
12 August 1842. Epigastric pain. Pulse 90. Skin hot.
Applic: Hirudines 2 to epigastrium.[2] *Two bottles soda water.*[3]
14 August 1842. Vin rubri 4 oz.[4]
15 August 1842. Pulse firm. Wine relished.
30 August 1842. Full diet.
2 October 1849. Dismissed cured.
Diagnosis in ward index – synocha.[5]   H. D. Littlejohn[6]

MARY ALEXANDER, aged 22
Farm servant
9 April 1849. Admitted ward 11.
States that for nearly eight years she has been subject to fits, occurring at intervals of three, four or five weeks. Is not aware of the length of time they last but is rendered unable to work for two or three days owing to pain of an aching, dull character in the head and back with general lassitude and great inclination to sleep. At the time she was first seized she suffered from a severe burn of the legs and this she refers to as the cause of her complaint.

---

[1] A public meeting on 3 August 1840 had led to the opening of the 'night asylum for the houseless poor' in Old Fishmarket Close This provided porridge at night, a bed and breakfast. People could thus sleep 'off stairs and streets.' Accommodation was for one night only although, as here, this was sometimes extended.

[2] 'Two leeches to be applied to epigastrium'.

[3] A refreshing drink.

[4] 'Red wine 4 ounces'.

[5] 'Synocha'. An old word meaning 'a continuous fever'.

[6] Littlejohn became first MOH for Edinburgh.

The last fit occurred five weeks ago and she had her head shaved, leeched and blistered for the subsequent symptoms which were unusually severe.

The fit is preceded by tingling and numbness of the fingers of the right hand. This gradually extends upwards to the shoulder and then passes down the left arm. She is sensible of this lasting for about ten minutes. Her brother, who is older than herself, is the only member of her family affected in a similar manner and his fits commenced when very young.

On examination found extended on her back, face slightly livid and teeth clenched. Eyes closed. Pupils dilated and acting very sluggishly. Arms and legs quite rigid. On forcibly bending them into any position they will retain it. Appears to be perfectly insensible to a severe pinch, but on dashing cold water on the face winking is produced. Respiration very slow and almost imperceptible. Pulse feeble, 63. This was the state on admission; no information could be obtained regarding the character attending the first seizure.

From this state she gradually recovered, the limbs becoming less rigid and cataleptic. In about three hours she was able to answer questions though in a very tedious and drawling manner. The pulse became fuller and quicker. Complains of great fatigue and drowsiness with considerable pain in the head.

Vespere. Hab. Ol: Ricini 1 ounce stat.[1]

11 April 1849. Head ordered to be shaved.

Applic. vesicatori vertici[2]

12 April 1849. Refused to allow head to be shaved and was dismissed in consequence.

HAMISH HENDERSON, aged 25

From Leith. A sailor.

8 June 1841. Admitted to surgical wards of Professor Syme.

This man has been treated in No. 5 Medical House for the last six weeks for scurvy, which he contracted on a merchant ship on her way from the East Indies. A short time before coming ashore

---

[1] 'Evening. To have one ounce of castor oil immediately'.

[2] 'Apply a blistering agent to crown of head.'

he sprained his right ankle which remained swollen and discoloured nearly two months afterwards.

The discolouration is now gone but there still exists some swelling and great tenderness on putting his foot to the ground. A bandage to be firmly applied. A few dark, livid spots still exist on the left leg.

23 July 1841. Dismissed cured.

JEAN MALCOLM, aged 5
Address not known
13 August 1849. Admitted to hospital. Healthy till last winter when she developed scarletina, and in the Spring, hooping cough [*sic*].[1]

Her mother, being a sick nurse, confided her to the keeping of a friend, 'who did not take proper care of her.' She was brought here chiefly on account of a small 'tumour' on the chest which had 'appeared suddenly' and, to the friend's knowledge, 'without cause.' She still complains of the cough which seems to have existed for upwards of two months.

On examination she presents some peculiarity in conformation of the chest, the sternum projecting very much, the last piece especially, so as to resemble a small tumour. Xiphoid cartilage scarcely developed.

Chest sounds well on percussion and sounds are healthy on auscultation. Hooping cough [*sic*] slight, especially at night, with recurrence.

Sumat olei morrhuae 1 drachm ter in die.[2]
25 August 1849. Dismissed relieved.

SUSAN MUIR, aged 33
Hume's Close. A hawker.
2 June 1844. Admitted to care of Professor Syme. When she was preparing to go to bed her cap accidentally caught fire from a candle standing on a table beside her. A shawl, which she had

---

[1] The spelling 'hooping cough', is also used by others, including a Dr West whose treatment for the disease is listed in Beasley's '*The Book of Prescriptions* (Henry Churchill, London, 1854).

[2] 'To have one drachm of cod liver oil three times a day.'

wound round her neck, also took fire and it was some time before assistance was got to extinguish the flames.

On examination the front of the neck and throat is found in a state of vesication. Some of the blisters have burst. Warm water dressings have been applied.

2 June 1844.(*vespere*).[1] In consideration of the situation of the burn she experiences considerable restriction in her breathing. To have half a grain of tartar emetic[2] in solution, with ten drops of the *Sol: Mur: Morph:*[3] three times daily.

3 June 1844. The difficulty in breathing is very much diminished.

5 June 1844. The difficulty in breathing is quite gone.

25 July 1844. Dismissed cured. Kelburne King

JOHN MILLER, aged 34
Market Street. A night policeman.
31 May 1841. Admitted to surgical wards of Professor Syme.

Admitted on account of haemorrhage from a small varicose ulcer of the size of a sixpence, situated on the lower part of the left shin. The veins of the leg are much enlarged and tortuous, and swell out on the patient assuming the erect posture. A poultice applied.

3 June 1841. A pin was today introduced under three of the veins in the upper part of the calf of the leg and secured by a twisted ligature.

7 June 1841. The swollen appearance and tortuosity of the veins is nearly gone and the sore, since the last report, has taken on a healing action. The pin causes very slight discolouration of the skin with slight tenderness in its neighbourhood.

[Notes incomplete]

---

[1] 'Vespere' means 'in the evening'.

[2] Tartar emetic is antimony potassium tartrate. Beasley describes it 'as the most certain and generally used preparation of antimony'. It had multiple uses, here probably being used to 'subdue inflammation'.

[3] Sol: Mur: Morph: is a solution of the hydrochlorate of morphia. This was known in Edinburgh and Dublin as *morphiae murias* (*British Pharmacopoeia*, 1867), because its preparation required long periods of maceration of the opium with water, ammonia solution and calcium chloride. The word '*murias*' was used by Horace to mean 'salt liquor, brine or pickle'

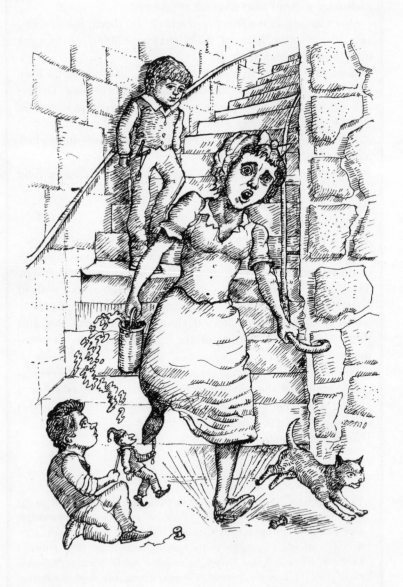

✣ 21 ✣

The Infirmary and Trauma

My bones are smitten asunder . . .

Psalm 42

This chapter is compiled from the case histories of people admitted to the Infirmary suffering from trauma of different kinds. It begins with what is probably the shortest case history in the ward journals.

RONALD McGUIRE
Tolbooth Wynd, Leith. A seaman.
Admission details not known. While walking along a plank with a sack on his back he fell and dislocated his hip. He was carried to the Royal Infirmary where it was reduced.

MARGARET WATERSTON, age unknown
Address and occupation unknown
17 June 1844. Admitted to surgical wards of Professor Syme. This morning she was coming down a stair carrying a pitcher of water when, supposing she had reached the ground although there still remained one step, she put out her foot incautiously and came violently down upon her heel. The ankle since very painful and she is unable to put it to the ground.

On examination the ankle is much swollen especially on the outer side. It has very much the appearance of a fracture of the fibula but, owing perhaps to the swelling, no crepitus can be perceived.

Warm fomentations to be applied.
21 June 1844. On examination the fibula is found fractured and the usual apparatus has been applied.
25 June 1844. Dismissed cured.

ELIZABETH DUNN, aged 23
Address not known
6 June 1848. Admitted to ward 11, Prof. Christison.

States that about five weeks ago received a severe blow on the crown of the head with the flat of the hand from a man who was tipsy. She was rendered stupid for about five minutes but did not fall. The same night there was some pain and swelling of the part. Next day the pain was very severe and has continued so ever since. Occasionally parts of the scalp swell and the pain is then greatly increased. The pain is always worst at night. It prevents her sleeping till morning or during the day.

On admission complains of severe pain over the forehead and vertex. The pain feels as if situated in the scalp. It is aggravated in the evening and during the night, becoming less towards morning when she generally gets some sleep. There is no tumefaction of the scalp and no perceptible irregularity of the bones of the cranium. Never has any startings [*sic*]. Vision and hearing not disordered.

Pulse 66, irregular, rather weak. Heart sounds distant and irregular. Percussion of chest and respiratory murmur natural. Catamenia[1] have not appeared for two months.

7 June 1848. Applic: hirudenis 8 temporibus.[2]
8 June 1848. Applic: cucurbitula cruenta et mitte sang: ad 10 oz.[3]
14 June 1848. A lotion for the left eye which is somewhat congested.
19 June 1848. Dismissed cured.   J. S.
but . . .

'A few days after being dismissed she was brought in to No. 10 by the police. She was insensible, having been knocked down and kicked in a horrid manner. She died comatose in two days.'
Sectio cadaveris

On examining the cranium a large flat clot of blood about three inches square was found between the dura mater and the cranium, over the course of the L. meningeal artery. Internal to this clot, and adherent to the dura mater, was a false membrane half a line

---

[1] 'Catamenia' means menstrual periods.
[2] 'Apply eight leeches to the temple'
[3] 'To be cupped using the scarifier and ten ounces of blood withdrawn.'

thick,[1] firm and of a reddish-yellow colour. This was evidently of some standing. The clot external to it had existed apparently for a few days only, probably since the date of the last injury. The meningeal artery could not be observed to be lacerated. No fracture of the cranial bones.'[2]

JOSEPH SEATON, aged 58
Borthwick's Close. A plasterer.
27 May 1844. Admitted to surgical wards of Professor Syme.

When going up a stair yesterday in a state of intoxication he fell down several steps and, being unable to rise, was carried to bed. It was observed that blood was flowing from the right ear. This morning blood continued to flow and he appeared to be quite insensible to what was going on about him, though sometimes he was very violent. It was noticed that his right arm was injured.

On examination the bleeding from the ear continues. It is impossible to get an answer to any question though he talks loudly and incoherently. The right humerus is found fractured about its middle but rather above it. There is no appearance of fracture of the bones of the cranium. The arm has been put up in the usual way with lateral pasteboard splints extending from the acromion and the axilla and grasping the elbow.

1 June 1844. Since admission he has remained in the state then noticed but today he is quieter. It is noted that he is quite deaf which he is said not to have been prior to the accident. He has taken hardly any food since his admission.

5 June 1844. He continues in much the same state. The swelling of the arm having sustained the fracture of the humerus is found to be considerably higher than was at first supposed. The arm is fixed to the ribs by a broad handkerchief.

5 July 1844. He has since admission been in a state of fatuity and perfectly deaf. Last night he was seized with a violent fit after which he died.   K.K.

---

[4] A 'line' was a unit of measurement equivalent to one-twelfth of an inch.
[5] This was an extradural haematoma.

MAY ELLIS, aged 20
Saxe Coburg Place. A servant.
10 May 1841. Admitted to surgical wards of Professor Syme on account of dislocation of both wrists from having fallen from a height of two storeys, pitching on the palms of her hands. The carpal bones were forced forwards and lay (on both sides) on the palmar aspect of the wrist.

They were easily reduced, there being very slight swelling. A paste board splint was placed along the palmar aspect of each forearm and hand, and secured by a bandage.

12 May 1841. Some pain and swelling around the wrists. Splints removed. Fomentations applied.

15 May 1841. Pain and swelling nearly gone. Wrists in good position. Splints reapplied

20 May 1841. Dismissed cured.   R. M.

IRENE CALLAGHAN, aged 46
A widow
28 November 1841. Admitted to Royal Infirmary. States that she left Ireland six weeks ago and has enjoyed good health up until a fortnight before admission when she was troubled with gravel and a cough. She says she has been much ill-used by her son-in-law and has even been knocked down by him while in a state of intoxication. She appears to have resorted to the Infirmary with the idea of getting out of his way rather than from any serious inconvenience resulting from disease.

On admission appears weak and feeble. Some sibilant and dry râles on both sides of chest. Has a cough with sputum. Complains of pain over whole body and particularly in arms and legs which appears to be of a rheumatic character.

℞ *Pulv: Colchicii.*[1] *Pulv: Doverii* [doses illegible].[2] *Misce et divide in pulv: 6. One ter in die.*[2]

[1] In addition to its 'almost specific power in relieving the paroxysm of gout', Beasley says colchicum's use 'has been extended to inflammatory affections generally. Its effects seem to be uncertain, and its use requires caution'.

[2] First prescribed by Dr Thomas Dover (1660-1742), Dover's powder is a preparation of opium, ipecacuanha root and potassium sulphate, 'used to induce sweating.' This and the colchicum powder were to be mixed and divided into six powders of which one was to be given three times a day.

1 December 1841. Much better. The pain has quite left her. Cough and expectoration however, very troublesome.

℞ *Sp: Aether Nit:* 2 drachms. *Vin Ipecac:* 1 drachm. *Tinct: Opii:* [illegible]. *Mist: Scillae* [illegible]. *Fiat mist. Sumat* 1 oz *ter in die.*[1]

5 December 1841. Cough and expectoration much relieved. Complains now of indigestion and a sense of weight and heaving in the epigastrium.

℞ *Ammon: Sesquicarb:* ½ drachm. *Tinct: Rhei:* 3 drachms. *Aqua: Menth: Pip:* 5½ oz. [?] *Fiat mist: 1 ounce ter in die.*[2]

25 December 1841. Dismissed cured.

HUGH IRONS, aged 54
Leith
21 June 1841. Admitted to surgical wards of Professor Syme.

The patient is stone deaf consequently a distinct account of his case cannot be obtained. Three or four days ago he fell the height of a few feet and struck his right side against a sharp corner. Great pain followed in the injured part and he had great difficulty of breathing, to which he had not formerly been subject.

He was bled from the arm and cupped in the loins.

On examination suffers great pain in taking a full inspiration or on pressure over the cartilages of the right lower ribs but more particularly over the eighth rib behind its angle. At this point a depression is felt but no crepitus detected.

A flannel roller was applied round the chest and twenty ounces of blood taken from the arm.

1 July 1841. Patient has made a good recovery. Dismissed cured.

R. M.

ROBERT THOMSON, aged 23
Canongate. A hawker.
9 June 1844. Admitted to surgical wards of Professor Syme.

---

[1] This combination was considered to be 'expectorant' and 'anodyne'.

[2] The mixture here used was for dyspepsia, although Beasley notes that 'the sesquicarbonate of ammonia, a synonym for carbonate of ammonia, is less irritant than the caustic ammonia'. Rheum is rhubarb. Aqua menth: pip: is aqua menthae piperitae or peppermint water.

About two o'clock of the morning of Thursday, a man with whom he was disputing at the top of a stair, pushed him and he fell down several steps. He has ever since complained of pain about the right shoulder and incapacity in raising the arm from the side.

On examination the clavicle is found fractured nearer its acromial than its sternal extremity. The fracture is oblique and the inner fragment projects above the outer.

The shoulders having been drawn backwards the fractured ends of the bone were placed in apposition and retained in their place by an apparatus consisting of a circular collar, padded with tow, put round each shoulder and firmly tied together behind with bandages. The arm is to be kept suspended in a sling.
29 June 1844. Dismissed cured.   K. K.

RICHARD ARBUCKLE, aged 37
High Street. A porter.
13 May 1841. Admitted to surgical wards of Professor Syme.

Admitted on account of fractures of the eighth and ninth ribs about half way between the angles and cartilages, sustained by a fall against a large stone on his left side. He has great pain on taking a deep breath and on coughing but no feverishness.
A flannel roller was firmly applied and rest enjoined.
℞ *Syrup Scillae* 1 oz. *Vin: Antim:* ½ oz. *Mucilaginis* 2½ oz. *Aqua* 4 oz. *Fiat mistura cujus sumat 1 drachm tussi urgenti.*[1]
17 May 1841. Still a good deal of sharp pain on taking a deep breath.
V S ad 20 ounces.[2] *Mistura continuatum.*[3]
19 May 1841. Feels quite well. Dismissed cured.   A. J. L

---

[1] The scilla in this mixture was used for its effect on cough. The antimony was to suppress inflammation. Three kinds of mucilage were in common use, gum acacia, starch and tragacanth. The latter, derived from astragalus, was considered a demulcent in coughs. It was also used to aid the suspension of insoluble powders in water. Here the mixture is to be used as needed for cough..

[2] V S means 'venesect', here to 20 ounces.

[3] 'Continue the mixture'.

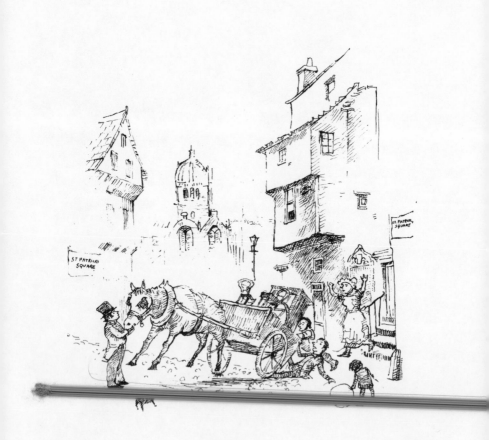

✤ 22 ✤

The Infirmary and the Horse

Do not trust the horse, Trojans!

VIRGIL, *Aeneid* 2,1.5

The following case histories are of people who, in one way or another, became too closely involved with horses. They come from the surgical ward journals of Mr Syme and include the unlucky Mrs Elizabeth Cairnie who had travelled up from the family farm near Stirling to the races at Musselburgh. The unusual stories of Turnbull and Robert Kerr and their horses come from medical wards and were told in an earlier chapter.

ELIZABETH CAIRNIE, aged 40
Parish of Blackford. Husband a farmer.
7 July 1848. While standing on a temporary erection, made for the purpose of witnessing the races at Musselburgh, it gave way and she was thrown on the ground a height of about six feet. Several loose rafters fell upon her right leg.

On examination the leg was found fractured above the lower fourth. Considerable swelling had taken place prior to her admission.

The usual apparatus was applied.
2 September 1848. Dismissed cured.

HAROLD THOMSON, aged 15
St Patricks' Square. A joiner.
27 May 1844. He states that a cart heavily laden with furniture, behind which he was walking, overbalanced and fell backwards, raising the horse which was dragging it into the air. On observing what was about to take place, he endeavoured to support the cart but, not having sufficient strength, was crushed below it. He does

---

not know exactly how he fell or what part came in contact with the ground first, but he thinks that his left leg was struck by the projecting beam at the end of the cart.

On examination the tibia is found fractured a little below its middle the fracture being nearly transverse but running a little obliquely from behind forwards and upwards. The fibula was broken a little higher up.

The fracture surfaces having been placed in apposition, lateral pasteboard splints were applied and secured by four looped bandages. The limb was then laid on its outer side and placed on a pillow, the knee being bent.

24 June 1844. Dismissed cured.

BRIAN SMITH, aged 24
Dumfries. A stableman.
23 July 1844. Admitted to surgical wards of Professor Syme. A week before admission, when riding on horseback, the horse shied and his right leg was brought violently into contact with the wheel of a cart. In the afternoon of the same day the leg became much swollen and very painful. Suppuration then took place and has since continued.

On examination a small opening is found on the skin over the right shinbone at its upper third. This leads into an extensive abscess extending between the skin and the periosteum and occupying about half the length of the leg.

25 July 1844. The opening above mentioned was today dilated.

17 August 1844. Dismissed cured.

AGNES MACPHERSON, aged 52
Fishmarket Close. Sells vegetables.
13 July 1844. Shortly before admission, while pursuing her calling in the vegetable market, she was knocked down by a horse which had started off and one of the wheels of a cart which it was dragging passed over her left leg. A crowd of people, who were on the spot at the time, being terrified by the accident, many of them ran over her as she lay on the ground.

On examination the left leg was found obliquely fractured

through the lower third of the tibia and upper third of the fibula. The displacement was very great and it has not been without considerable difficulty that the fragments were got into apposition. Several of the ribs on the right side have been fractured near their cartilages. The shock seems to have been very great and she still laboured under it when admitted, the extremities being very cold and the pulse hardly perceptible. She is quite unable to give an account of herself.

The leg has been put up in the usual manner and a flannel bandage applied round the chest. Warm water bottles have been placed about the legs and body.

13 July 1844. (*vespere*) Remains almost pulseless but complains very much of pain. The skin over the seat of the fracture is of a dark colour. To have two ounces of whisky.

14 July 1844. Pulse still feeble. Dark colour of the leg extending. Continue whisky.

15 July 1844. She is better today but pulse weak, 120.

18 July 1844. She passed a very restless night and today her breathing is hurried, the pulse hardly to be felt and her face of a yellowish colour. Much thirst and pain about the chest. The right Os Innominatum is fractured, the upper part of the ilium being quite mobile, but she has no pain in the part.

19 July 1844. She has continued to sink since yesterday and she died at 8 pm. Kelburne King

ALLAN GLEN, aged 32
Address unknown. A labourer
13 June 1844. This morning about 6 am the wheel of a cart, in which was a stone weighing 7 tons, passed over his left leg. The accident happened at Carfrae Mill, about twenty miles from town and he was immediately put in a cart and brought here. He arrived about 6 pm. [i.e. twelve hours later]

On examination a wound is found about the middle of the leg but nearer the knee on its anterior surface. It is about two inches in length and the soft parts about it are very much contused, as indeed is the whole of the calf. On passing the finger into the wound several large pieces of the tibia were found lying quite detached from their connections. These were removed. The tibia is fractured in two other places, one immediately below its head and the other about four inches above the ankle joint. The head of the fibula is felt dislocated upwards and outwards but it does not appear to have been fractured.

He is in a state of great collapse, his extremities cold, his pulse barely perceptible and his faculties obscured.

Hot bottles were put about him and he got two ounces of whisky.

Mr Syme saw him about an hour after he was admitted and though his pulse was still very feeble he was advised to submit to amputation at the thigh. To this, however, he would not submit.

14 June 1844. He continues still in the same low condition, his pulse is weak and quick, p. 118, and his mental faculties are still slow and as if oppressed. The dorsum of the foot and the neighbourhood of the wound are of dark bluish colour as if gangrene was coming.

15 June 1844. His pulse is not quite so feeble today though still very compressible. His faculties are somewhat abolished. The appearances of gangrene are today more decided about the margin of the wound. He is said to have been a man of dissipated habits.

16 June 1844. The gangrene had extended considerably this morning and he was in a very feeble condition. He continued to sink till 2 pm when he died. Kelburne King

MURRAY MASON, aged 16
Water of Leith. A carter.
24 June 1841. A few hours before his admission a horse, which he was leading, took fright and struck him with its forefoot on the back of the head and the shoulder.

The back of the head is slightly cut and the shoulder very bruised.

Head shaved and cold applied.
4 July 1841. Dismissed cured.

HUGH COCHRANE, age unknown
Liberton parish. A carter.
3 July 1841. Admitted to surgical wards of Professor Syme on account of an injury of the head sustained about half-an-hour previously. He was in a state of insensibility and a correct account of the accident could not be ascertained. It was stated, however, that he had fallen, while intoxicated, from a cart which he was driving and that one of the wheels passed over his right shoulder and head.

On examination he was in a state of collapse, the pulse small and weak, the extremities cold and with blood issuing from both ears and nostrils. The head was shaved and a contusion discovered a little above and in front of the left ear but no fracture or depression detected. The right clavicle was fractured obliquely about the middle and he complained on handling the part as on pressing on the injured part of the head. Pupils contracted.

Cold was applied to the head, warm bottles to the extremities and a turpentine enema was immediately given which however was not retained. Figure-of-eight bandage to the shoulders.

About two o'clock sensibility had considerably improved and the pulse had risen though still weak.
4 July 1841. More sensible but still answers questions very incoherently. There is a considerable degree of strabismus. Pulse 80, not strong. The turpentine enema has been retained and this morning he has vomited a large quantity of fluid having a strong odour of turpentine. In the evening the pulse was stronger. There was no pain in the head but considerable drowsiness.
℞ To have ¼ gr. of tartrate of antimony every two hours.[1]
5 July 1841. Sensibility improved. Squinting continues. The swelling of the head has diminished and the presence of a depression of the skull is suspected. Pulse 94, full. He was cupped to twelve ounces and the antimonials continued. Bowels unopened.
℞ Two drops of croton oil and to be repeated if necessary.[2]

---

[1] While antimonials were used as anti-inflammatory agents, the tartrate of antimony here was possibly being used as a 'contra-stimulant' or 'revulsive'. In this use Beasley says 'an effect is sought on one organ by the substance's action on another.'

[2] Croton oil is very toxic. Used as a laxative in the unconscious, the dose being two drops placed on the tongue.

6 July 1841. Much the same as yesterday. Vomiting occasionally. Bowels were not acted on by four drops of croton oil but have today been freely evacuated by a purgative enema. The depression appears more distinct today. The drowsiness continues.

8 July 1841. Complains today of more pain in the head and is more drowsy. Pulse 100.

Venae sectio ad [illegible]. *Continue antimonials and purgatives.*[1]

15 July 1841. Has made gradual improvement since last night. The squint, however, continues and he remains rather drowsy. Pulse natural.

8 August 1841. Is now free of complaint. The squint remains and the eyelid of the right eye slightly droops. Dismissed cured.

[1] 'Bleed to [amount].'

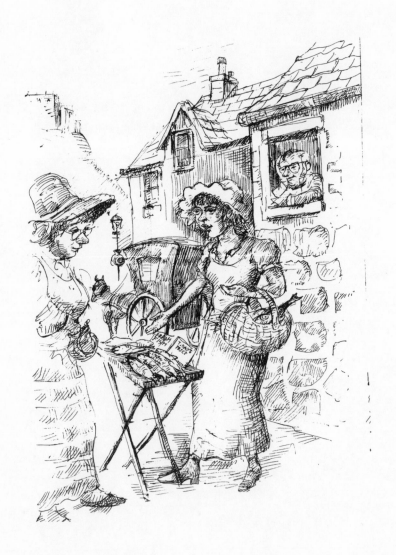

23

The Infirmary and the Fishing Industry

It's no' fish ye're buying – it's men's lives.
SCOTT, *The Antiquary*, 1816

'The quantity of fresh herrings purchased, during the period they are in season, in the High Street of the Old Town is immense; and during the many Saturday nights when we made our observations, we saw great quantities of them bought with avidity, apparently by the very poorest class of inhabitants. Some of the fishwomen occasionally take up a station at the 'Lazy Corner' with the remains of the fish offered before in the day's market, or perhaps hawked up and down the streets. This sort of stuff is offered very cheap, in fact at almost any price, the object being to get the creels emptied as soon as possible.' This extract, taken from *Low Life in Victorian Edinburgh* by a 'Medical Gentleman' referred to earlier, reflects the great days of the Scottish herring industry. Vast numbers were caught as the fish moved round the coast each summer. With an equally good supply of beef and mutton available from the market at the Falkirk Tryst to the west of Edinburgh, and oatmeal, barley and vegetables in plenty, an excellent diet was available, at a reasonable cost, for the people of the city. A reasonable cost was, however, still too much for many as Infirmary records of malnourished patients show.

The two fishermen, Darroch and Paterson, whose stories are told elsewhere in this book, were both Shetlanders. They were injured on their separate boats and admitted eventually to the Infirmary. Another fisherman, John Ross from the Shore, Leith, thought that his chronic respiratory illness had begun when he was 'cast away amongst the ice in the Davis Strait.' The less dramatic stories of others who worked with fish are told below.

COLIN MCANDREW, aged 42
A labourer. Kilmuir, Isle of Skye.
18 July 1884. Admitted to surgical wards of Professor Syme. A cask filled with herrings, which he was rolling up a declivity, slipped from his hold and struck against his left leg.

On examination there is considerable swelling about two inches above the anterior [*sic*] malleolus but no fracture seems to have taken place.
24 July 1884. Dismissed cured.   Kelburne King

CHRISTINA AHERNE, aged 40
Grassmarket. Originally Co. Monaghan, Ireland. Married.
27 August 1848. Admitted to ward 11.

Fourteen days ago caught cold while gathering shellfish. Since then has had considerable obstinate cough with some shortness of breath. Eight days ago a profuse spit appeared. Has never ceased her employment.

On admission there is a feeling of weight over right side of chest. Much cough, some dyspnoea. On percussion the chest sounds well in all parts. On auscultation, coarse mucous râles in all parts of chest. Expiration prolonged with sonorous vibration. There is some subcrepitous râle in lower left chest posteriorly. The heart sounds are natural. Pulse 96.
28 August 1848. Applicatur vesicatorum 4x4 pectoris dextro.[1]
11 September 1848. Dismissed relieved

PATRICIA CUMMING, aged 54
Burntisland. A fish-woman.
10 June 1841. Admitted to surgical wards of Professor Syme.

Admitted on account of a neglected whitlow of the right forefinger. Pricked the point of the finger six weeks ago with the point of a dirty fish hook. Great pain and swelling of the point of the finger immediately followed and gradually extended upwards. Poultices were applied and after three weeks an incision was made and a quantity of thick matter evacuated. Sloughing of the extremity of the finger followed and sinuses formed at various parts of the finger.

---

[1] 'To have a blister, four inches by four inches, applied to right side of chest.'

On examination the whole finger is found much swollen and three sinuses lead down to the bone at different parts. The soft parts have sloughed from the extremity of the finger and the distal phalanx is exposed.

17 June 1841. The finger was today removed, along with the head of the metacarpal bone, by a flap from the radial and ulnar sides of the digit.

19 June 1841. Some redness and swelling of the hand and at a circumscribed spot over the tendon of the biceps. Bandages removed and warm fomentations applied, the edges of the wound being kept in apposition by adhesive straps.

5 July 1841. Dismissed cured.

MARY O'MALLEY, aged 14
Grassmarket, originally Co. Leitrim, Ireland. A fish crier.
25 August 1848. Admitted to ward 11.

Six days ago, after being occupied all day selling fish on the streets, felt a sharp pain in the left side, not constant nor severe on taking a deep breath. Next day the pain was constant but not so sharp. Loss of appetite, great thirst. Great difficulty in breathing, even in bed. Since then confined to bed and has also felt a little on the right side. Three months ago she had a somewhat similar attack though not so severe and she continued at her occupation. Pain was then first on the right and then on the left.

On admission the countenance is flushed and oppressed, the skin hot, red and dry. No appetite, much thirst. Complains of dull pain in lower part of left side, none on right. There is considerable dyspnoea and some cough which causes pain in left side. Pulse 120.

On percussion the left side sounds well above the fourth rib in front. Below that it gets duller. Behind it sounds well as low as the middle of the scapula below which it rapidly becomes dull being completely dull in the lower third. The right side, behind, sounds pretty well. In front sounds well to an inch below the nipple. Hepatic dullness extends further up than natural

On auscultation the respiratory murmur below the left clavicle is puerile. Immediately above the nipple and around it subcrepitous râle is heard. Below this, and extending into the axilla, fine crepitations are heard in some parts with tubular respiration in all parts. Behind there are the same sounds and there is a friction sound. On the right side there are fine crepitations and slight friction, with subcrepitous râle behind.

She was bled on admission to 12 oz. which caused some faintness. It relieved the dyspnoea considerably and diminished the strength but not the frequency of the pulse. She had also: ℞ *Antimonii tartari* 4 grains. *Aquae cinnamon. Aqua fontis.* of each, 4 oz. Make a solution. *Sumat 1 ounce secunda quaque hora.*[1]

30 August 1848. Takes a full breath without pain and feels much better. Blood very lusty [*sic*].

Continuatim mistura.[2]

11 September 1848. Dismissed cured.

---

[1] This mixture of antimony in cinnamon water and 'spring water' was to be given in a dose of one ounce every second hour.

[2] 'Continue the mixture.'

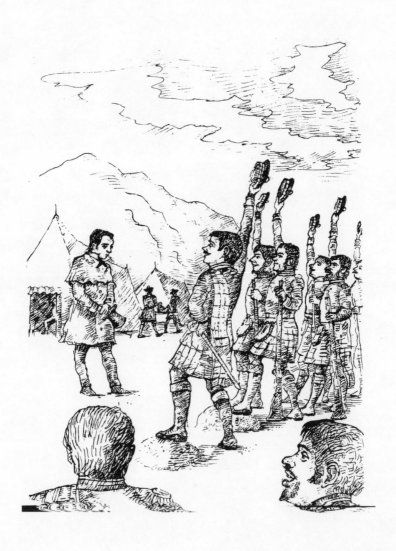

❧ 24 ❧

Another Surgeon

Before undergoing a surgical operation,
arrange your temporal affairs; you may live!

AMBROSE BIERCE

Richard McKenzie was born in 1821 and twenty years later was a junior doctor in Professor Syme's wards. He was keen to succeed in surgery and was able to work well with Syme. He was not, however, allowed to extend his clerkship with the Professor beyond the usual maximum of two years. Many of the case histories he wrote up in the ward journals of wards 2, 5 and 6 are to be found in this book. Two are recorded below. Both show his skill in writing a clinical history. The second case describes the rugged management of an orthopaedic problem in the days before X-rays and anaesthetics.

ALEXANDER DARROCH, aged 17
A fisherman from Shetland.
20 May 1841. Admitted to surgical wards of Professor Syme on account of an aneurysm of the femoral artery immediately below the situation where the sartorius crosses the vessel. Three months ago, while engaged in cutting a stick, his hand slipped and the knife entered the inner side of the left thigh a little below its middle. A large jet of blood immediately took place but was arrested in about two minutes by the application of four half-crowns over the wound secured by a firm bandage.

The wound healed in a few days and he felt nothing remarkable till eight days after when he perceived a thrilling sensation in the part which increased every day. Fourteen days after the injury he first perceived a pulsating tumour in the region of the wound about the size of a small hen's egg. This excited no alarm and no treatment was employed till about one week ago when, the tumour having gradually increased, he applied to a

---

surgeon who applied a flannel roller tightly round the thigh and sent him to the hospital.

On admission the limb was slightly oedematous and he complained of it having been cold ever since the application of the bandage. The tumour was found to be immediately on the lower edge of the sartorius, having a strong pulsatory movement, of the size of a goose egg but not very distinctly defined. The sac is found to be easily emptied by pressure, either over the tumour or on the artery in the groin, and no trace of the tumour can be perceived when thus emptied. A loud bruit is heard on the application of the ear to the tumour. The patient seems to have a strong constitution and his health is good.

To have the low diet of this hospital.

26 May 1841. A ligature was today applied to the femoral artery in the triangular space in the usual manner. One small vessel was divided and tied during the operation. Pulsation was completely arrested in the sac. Wound dressed by suture and a compress on each side, with a bandage.

27 May 1841. Slept well and has little or no constitutional disturbance. Limb of perfectly natural temperature and the seat of no uneasy sensations. Sac decidedly shrunk in size and feels firm as if filled by coagulum. Low diet to be continued. To have a saline purgative at bedtime.

28 May 1841. Was a little feverish last night. An antimonial solution[1] was ordered and six ounces of black draught[2] to be given this morning. Today his skin is cool and he feels well.

30 May 1841. Has been quite well since last report. The tumour is shrinking daily in size. It is now scarcely perceptible to the eye and free of all pulsation.

7 June 1841. Wound nearly closed with very slight discharge. The tumour is now not perceptible to the eye and feels a small firm

---

[1] Antimonial preparations were considered to be anti-inflammatory

[2] The 'black draught' consisted of senna (in two forms: an infusion with ginger and a tincture), tincture of jalapa, magnesium sulphate and ginger syrup. According to Beasley the black draught of most hospitals, was given exactly as in this case i.e. at the beginning of an inflammatory process and some hours after a preliminary aperient in order 'to accelerate its operation.'

mass entirely devoid of pulsation. Low diet continued. Strict rest enjoined.

14 June 1841. Ligature separated today with a slight pull. Wound nearly healed.

23 June 1841. Dismissed cured.

TOM PATERSON, aged 17
Cranston parish. A carter.

30 June 1841. Admitted to surgical wards of Professor Syme. Nine weeks ago fell out of a cart backwards and pitched, as he says, on the left elbow. He instantly lost the power of flexion of the joint. A surgeon to whom he applied told him the arm was broken and the elbow out of joint. Extension was accordingly made by six persons but reduction was not affected. A bandage was applied and the arm retained in a sling. He, however, possessed no motion in the joint nor has any improvement since taken place.

All the signs of a lateral dislocation of the elbow are present. Little or no motion is present in the joint, the hand and forearm are pronated and the inner condyle of the humerus projects inwards and feels thickened. The finger can be pressed into the fossa on the posterior aspect of the humerus. The olecranon is felt projecting on the outer condyle and the head of the radius is prominent. The external lateral ligament is stretched. Considerable power of pronation and supination is possessed.

3 July 1841. An attempt at reduction by powerful extension was made today. The ends of the bones were felt to yield considerably but reduction was not effected.

12 July 1841. Dismissed with advice.   R. McKenzie

THE CRIMEA

On 4 November 1848, McKenzie was appointed an assistant surgeon to the Infirmary and it is recorded that he was 'beginning to rival his master, Syme, in surgical skill.' But now his ambition led him to a critical decision. He knew that Sir George Ballingall would retire in a few years from the Chair of Military Surgery in Edinburgh University. McKenzie set out to succeed him, and to do so, he knew he would require surgical experience in the field.

This led him to be an early volunteer for service in the Crimean War. He left Britain in June 1854, joining the 79th Highland Regiment at Varna on the Black Sea coast of Bulgaria. There was much cholera in the Army before it embarked for the invasion of the Crimea but little surgery to be done. It was now thirteen years since he had treated Tom Paterson and anaesthesia had been introduced in Edinburgh. McKenzie wrote to J. Y. Simpson in Edinburgh, saying that he 'hoped there would be abundant supplies of chloroform' for his soldier patients.

He landed in time to take part in the battle of Alma, and in a few hours of hectic surgery, did thirty-two 'capital' operations including two amputations at the hip. Next day the regiment asked permission to give their surgeon three cheers in recognition of his work.

Two days later he was dead, struck down by cholera. He was thirty-three years old.

His death caused a vacancy for an assistant surgeon at Edinburgh Royal Infirmary which was eventually filled, in 1856, by Joseph Lister, Syme's son-in-law. Richard McKenzie's story has an ironic ending. Shortly after Sir George Ballingall retired as professor of military surgery in 1855, the Regius chair was abolished.

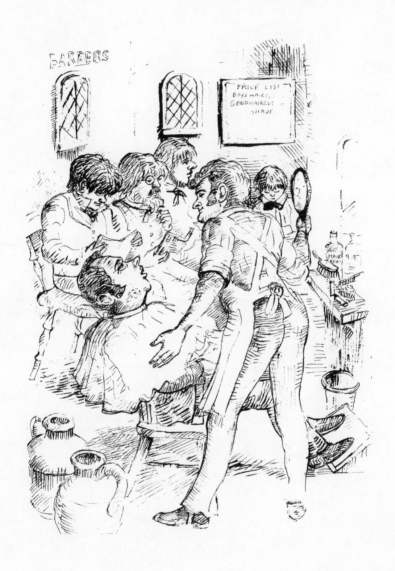

❧ 25 ❧

A Success Story

Out, damned spot! Out, I say!

SHAKESPEARE, *Macbeth*

Doctors working in the 1840s used a wide range of medicines but only a few were significantly effective. The management of diseases of the skin was much more successful, many patients leaving the hospital genuinely improved. There was no specialist skin department in the Royal Infirmary until 1884. Before then patients with skin problems were looked after by the general physicians, from whose ward journals the following case notes come.

JANE WADDELL, aged 30

Potter Row. A sempstress.

Admission date unknown. A single woman. Lives, and has lived for two years, as mistress to a man. Complains of no pain but of a skin eruption over whole body and limbs. States that this eruption began in the Spring, six months ago as she thinks but not positive. It commenced as itchiness and redness, then appeared yellow blisters which she constantly scratched and caused to bleed. She is positive that it commenced as small yellow blisters from the first.

Now the eruption extends over the entire body and limbs, more frequent on the back and arms. Seldom seen on the front of the body and legs. It consists of isolated pustules which have broken and formed ulcerated surfaces irregular in size from a pea to a four pence piece, most oval, some few circular. The ulcers are mostly dark livid brown covered by a thin transparent scab and seated on a patch of erythema. Irregularly scattered, not grouped. Numerous scratch marks mixed in with a number of recent flea bites. No vesicles anywhere. Skin soft and moist.

Pulse 74, natural. Catamenia[1] absent for fifteen months. Says she is not certain whether she is pregnant. Says positively she has never had syphilis nor any vaginal discharge.

26 July. 18—. ℞ *Hab: quotidia- balneum alkalinum cum soda carbonat:* 4 oz.[2]

℞ *Potass: Carb:* ½ drachm. *Tinct: Gent: Co:*[3] 1 oz. *Inf: Gent: Co:* 7 oz. *Fiat mist. Sumat* 1 oz *ter quotidae.*

4 August. Dismissed cured.

Index of ward journal gives diagnosis as ecthyma.[4]

MARION CORBETT, aged 14
Address unknown.
27 December 1849. Admitted to ward 11.

States that she has had an eruption upon her scalp for two years which has much annoyed her from the continual itching. Otherwise has enjoyed good health. About a fortnight since, she says, she caught 'the itch' from sleeping with another girl who had it, and that afterwards she communicated it to her sister who is also in the ward.

On admission the hair of the head is all matted together. On her hands, especially about the root of the fingers, arms and chest wall are seen numerous vesicles. On the chest the eruption is chiefly papular, and at the roots of the fingers and between them, pustules are seen in consequence of her scratching them. In other respects she is perfectly healthy.

The head is to be poulticed and lard applied to the eruption on the hands, arms and chest.

5 January 1850. The head has been shaved and now is quite clean. The surface looks red and raw where the scabs were, with little depression in it. The hands and arms are looking better. Ordered the head be kept moist with cod liver oil.

---

[1] Catamenia is an old word for menstrual periods.
[2] 'To have, four times a day, an alkaline bath with four ounces sodium carbonate'.
[3] Gentian was 'used internally as an antiseptic'. (Beasley) 'To have one ounce of this mixture three times a day.'
[4] Ecthyma is a pyogenic skin infection caused by beta-haemolytic streptococci and going on to ulceration and healing with scar formation.

℞ *Tinct: Ferri: Mur:* 1 drachm. *Tinct: Gent: Co:* 1 oz. *Infus:* 5 oz. *Sumat* ½ oz. *ter die.*[1]

5 February 1850. The eruption is quite gone from the head and limbs. Dismissed cured.

Diagnosis – tinea favosa and scabies.[2]

PATRICK O'CONNOR, aged 47

Labourer

17 March 1848. Admitted to hospital. On the 15th January, having been shaved by a country barber on the 6th, he felt great itching of his chin and observed some pimples over the part. These were accompanied by great heat which caused him to rub the part. They gradually spread over the whole chin and throat so far as was covered with hair and they ascended amongst his beard almost as high as the malar bones, spreading over his upper lip.

On examination small lumps observed over the part. They are about the size of a split pea, of firm consistence and a red colour, none containing pus.

℞ *Pulv: Jalapa 1 drachm. Calomelanos* 4 grains. *Ft Pulv:* [dose illegible].[3]

20 March 1848. Face to be painted each morning with *Tinct: Iodini.*

1 May 1848. Has become quite well of the sycosis under the use of Donovan's Solution but became affected with otitis which was associated with an abscess of the tympanum. Today there is an erysipelatous inflammation from the right ear over the right side of the face and forehead.[4]

℞ *Tinct: Opii* 1 oz. *Acet: Plumb:* 2 drachms. *Aqua* 10 oz. *Ft: lotio Abradatum capitis.*[5]

2 May 1848. Erysipelas rather extending but not very severe.

---

[1] This is a combination of iron and gentian root, from which an infusion was made and given, according to Beasley, as a 'tonic'.

[2] Tinea favosa is a fungal skin infection of ringworm type. 'favosa' means 'of honeycomb appearance'.

[3] A powder of jalapa, which is a purgative and the multi-use mercurial, calomelanos.

[4] Donovan's Solution is a mixture of arsenious and mercuric iodides.

[5] 'Shave the head and apply the lead and opium lotion.'

4 May 1848. Erythema crossing from ear to left side of face. Face to be dusted with flour.

6 May 1848. Erysipelas now fading on right and not extending on left. Continue medicament.

22 May 1848. Dismissed cured.

Diagnosis – sycosis barbae.

FRANCES CAMERON, aged 15

Cowgate (initially from Dunfermline). A servant.

30 August 1849. Admitted to hospital. Was in good health until the end of 1847 when she was admitted to hospital with fever. Six months ago she observed some red spots upon her legs preceded by some constitutional disturbance. Spots began at the knees, spreading over the rest of the legs. They next appeared at the elbows from which they spread as in the legs.

On examination appears very healthy. Complains of great itchiness from the eruption. Both extremities present the characteristics of lepra,[1] the larger patches near the knees and elbows. Towards the shoulders and wrists the eruption presents more the appearance of the second stage while those at elbow and knee are covered in scales. The largest patch is some inches in length.[1]

Apply Unguentum Picis.[2]

[1] Initially 'lepra' was a descriptive word for a particular type of skin lesion. Its use was then broadened to mean the disease psoriasis. After the middle of the nineteenth century it came to mean only the disease leprosy. Another patient, Aileen Cooper, who was a washerwoman, admitted to the Infirmary around this time, had lesions which were described as follows: 'The greater part of the body and limbs covered with lepra, most severe on the inferior extremities, especially the joints. Of the upper limbs the left is more affected than the right. On the chest it seems mixed with prurigo. The size of the eruption varies from that of a fourpenny piece to that of the hand. It presents the ordinary characters of lepra vulgaris but in many of the patches the centre is as hard and elevated as the circumference. The largest patch, over the right ilium is redder and more cracked than the others, resembling psoriasis inveterata. Mixed with the others are some small spots of psoriasis guttata. Over the joints, especially the knees where the eruption is worst, she complains of great pain upon motion.' She also was treated with tar ointment but less successfully.

[2] Unguentum picis is tar ointment, 'made, largely in North America, by the slow combustion of various species of pine' (Beasley).

27 September 1849. Has been much improved by use of this ointment.

13 October 1849. Dismissed cured.

4 December 1849. Readmitted. Eruption began to reappear about fourteen days after dismissal and has increased since.

Apply Unguentum Picis bis in die.

22 December 1849. Dismissed cured.

Diagnosis – psoriasis

ARTHUR NEWMAN, aged 22

Semple Street, initially Durham. A labourer.

1 July 1845. Admitted to hospital. Of florid complexion, robust and strongly marked with the smallpox. Says he is at work at present on the Union Canal but has been several years in England. Is in good employment and living on good food.

He has entered the house on account of a cutaneous eruption of five months duration which, he says, came out immediately after a wetting which he got by falling into the canal when it was covered with ice. Both arms and legs are affected. The affected portions of skin are rough and scabrous from adherent laminated scales. There is considerable itching. Where the scabs are abraded a number of red points are seen which exude a considerable quantity of serous fluid. A few scattered solitary vesicles, inclining to the pustular appearance, are seen on the arms and upper part of body. None of these appear on the legs and none between the fingers.

He has had medical advice before coming in and, in particular, mentions having made trial of various astringents, of pitch ointment and of washes of buttermilk.

24 July 1845. Since last report has been using the alkaline wash.[1] The right leg is almost free from eruption. On the surface here and there are patches of chronic eruption. On the left leg this is more intense causing slight induration in patches.

℞ *Ung: Picis*

4 August 1845. Dismissed relieved.   W. T. Gairdner

Diagnosis in ward journal – chronic eczema.

---

[1] 'Alkaline wash'. Probably a solution of sodium bicarbonate.

UNUSUAL CASES FROM THE JOURNALS: V

JOHN EVANS, aged 30
Carmarthenshire. A currier on the tramp.
18 August 1848. Admitted to surgical wards of Professor Syme.

Was admitted yesterday morning to No. 8 on account of a burn which he is understood to have received in consequence of having sat down on a fireplace in a state of intoxication. He however left the House shortly after admission and was brought back by his friends this morning.

There is a very extensive severe burn of both hips, the inside of both thighs and the point of the penis.
30 August 1848. The burn was dressed with warm water and latterly with a solution of sulphate of zinc. It healed quickly except a portion about the size of the palm of a man's hand which cicatrised more slowly. It is now almost quite healed and he is today dismissed cured.   K. K.

WILLIAM MURRAY, aged 19
Lochearnhead. A farm servant.
7 September 1849. For three months he has been affected with difficulty of breathing. No other symptom was present although he has been unable to work for that time.

On admission appears perfectly healthy and on examination nothing abnormal was detected except the slowness of his pulse which was forty-five. Dr Christison, however, discovered a slight roughness with the first sound of the heart. He was ordered:
Chloroform 1 drachm. *Tinct: Card: Co:* 7 drachms. *Solve. Sumat* 1 drachm *ex aqua ter in die.*[1]
24 September 1849. Dismissed cured.   A. Christison[2]
Diagnosis in ERI admissions register – ? aortic disease.

[1] Chloroform, recently introduced as an anaesthetic, was now being used also as a medicine, here possibly as an 'antispasmodic'. The cardamom was to improve the taste. One drachm of the mixture was to be given in water three times a day.

[2] The son of Professor Christison.

JAMES JACK, aged 17
Leith. An ironmonger.
17 June 1844. Admitted to surgical wards of Professor Syme. He was dragging a wheelbarrow on which was a turner's lathe. While descending a steep street the weight behind became too great for his strength and he was rolled over, the wheel passing over his right arm.

On examination the right humerus is found fractured a little below the middle of the shaft and there is considerable bruising of the upper part of the forearm.

Lateral pasteboard splints have been applied in the usual way.
27 July 1844. Dismissed cured. K.K.

CHARLES DONOVAN, aged 55
Blackfriar's Wynd, initially from Ireland
21 June 1841. Admitted to surgical wards of Professor Syme.

Admitted with stricture of the urethra of twelve years standing, the result of a gonorrhoea [*sic*]. Shortly after the first appearance he was treated by Mr Liston and after eight months treatment the urethra was dilated to its full size. Contraction gradually took place and four years ago he was admitted into Mr Syme's wards when the smallest size bougie was passed with difficulty. In seven weeks No 6 was passed but the patient was obliged, from circumstances, to return home. Since that time the stricture has again gradually returned.
23 June 1841. A passed with some difficulty.
28 June 1841. B, C, D and F passed comparatively easily.
1 July 1841. Nos. 1, 2, 3 and 4 passed.
8 July 1841. Nos. 3 and 4 passed. Two hours after, he had a severe rigor followed by heat of skin and general feverishness. He was immediately put into a warm bath and antimonials given.
10 July 1841. Patient again quite well. The stream is also much improved.
21 July 1841. Dismissed cured.

HENRY SIMON, aged 10
Dunbar.
Admitted to surgical wards of Professor Syme, 3/6/1844.

3 June 1844. About three months ago, after his having had several severe rigors, his right foot became swollen, red and painful. Poultices were applied to the foot and in the course of a week an opening was found in front of the internal malleolus from which a quantity of purulent matter was discharged. The pain disappeared. The redness and swelling of the posterior part of the foot and heel still remained and occasionally abscesses formed and opened at different points about ankle and knee during which the pain returned. Of late he has become much emaciated, his appetite has fallen off and he has become much debilitated.

On examination the foot is much swollen behind the ankle and the skin is red. Numerous sinuses exist on each side of the heel and over the ankle joint, into which a probe introduced passes distinctly into the substance of the bone. The ankle is stiff and any attempt to move it or to rest the weight of the body on that foot is attended with pain.

5 June 1844. The foot was today removed at the ankle joint. A thin plate of the tibia and the internal and external malleoli were removed with it. Six arteries required ligation. On examination the calcaneum was found carious throughout and the anterior surface of the ankle joint was also carious.[1]

8 June 1844. The greater part of the edges of the wound have adhered by first intention. Only a little pus in the discharge from the inner side of the wound.

20 June 1844. The wound is now quite healed except a very small portion.

2 July 1844. Dismissed cured.   K.K.

---

[1] This sounds like a 'Syme's amputation' and may have been one of the series of fourteen he reported in 1844.

KATHLEEN FLANAGAN, aged 33
303 Cowgate, formerly of Co. Cavan, Ireland
Husband a labourer
29 September 1848. Admitted to ward 11. Twelve days ago was seized with severe haemorrhage and the day after was delivered of a dead child, three months old. States that for three days after, the flooding continued. On the fourth day after delivery was seized with severe rigors followed by acute pain in the hypogastrium.

The countenance is pale, shrunk and expressive of great suffering. Hands and feet cold. She lies on her back with the thighs drawn upwards and flexed on the abdomen. On applying pressure over the uterine region she complains of great pain. The uterus appears enlarged. On examining *per vaginam* the parts within are hot and painful and the neck and os uteri are greatly swollen. The secretions, namely the milk and the lochia, are checked. Bowels not opened for two days. Pulse 126, soft. Respirations hurried.

℞ *Enema communis cum terebinth* ½ o*unce*.[1]

℞ *Vini oz. 4 and oz. 8 of beef tea.*[2] *A turpentine embrocation was applied to the abdomen.*[3]

30 September 1848. Pulse 95, hardly perceptible. No pain on pressure in uterine area. Answers questions in a confused manner. Lochia returned this morning. Bowels opened by injection.[4]

Ordered *Vini* oz. 8 with beef tea.

℞ *Ammon: carb:* gr. 36. *Mist: camphorae oz. 12.*[5]

Sumat [? dose] *quis ter hora* [?]

30 September 1848. (*vespere*) She died.

Diagnosis – puerperal fever

---

[1] The 'usual' enema [probably mucilage of starch] with ½ ounce turpentine.

[2] The prescription of [red] wine was common when the illness was thought to be terminal.

[3] An embrocation was a liquid to rub on the body to relieve pain.

[4] 'By injection' is from 'injiciatur enema', and thus simply means an enema.

[5] Mist: camphor was a synonym for camphor water. This mixture used empirically for 'prostration.'

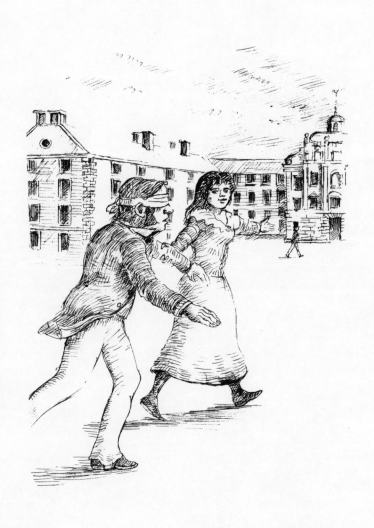

❧ 26 ❧

Four Eye Cases

He had but one eye, and the popular prejudice
runs in favour of two.

DICKENS, *Nicholas Nickleby*

Dr Duncan carried out a cataract operation in the Royal Infirmary in
June 1844. He asked the board to refund to him the cost of 'a pair of
strong spectacles'. To save delay for the patient, Duncan had paid for
them initially himself as he had done in the past. Before such specialist
care was available the Infirmary's general surgeons had done what
they could for people with eye problems. The following cases are
taken from the ward journals of the 1840s.

FAITH SUTHERLAND, aged 20
Muckhart. A servant.
8 July 1841. Admitted to surgical wards of Professor Syme with
ulceration of the cornea of the left eye about its centre. There is a
good deal of opacity round the ulcer and several red vessels are
seen running over the corneal surface. The complaint commenced
about six weeks ago without assignable cause. Scarification and
blistering have been employed.
℞ *Vin: Opii* ½ oz. *Aqua* ½ oz. *Nitri: Argent:* 2 grains. *Solve et misce
Fiat collyrium.*[1] *Cucurb: cruent: ad* 12 ounces i*n nucha.*[2] *Emplast:
colloc. post aur.*[3]

[1] A collyrium is an eyewash, here containing silver nitrate.
[2] '*Cucurb: cruent:*' means '*cucurbitula cruenta*' which means 'a cupping glass
with the scarificator'. A scarificator is an instrument for making several
incisions simultaneously. The instruction here is 'use the cupping glass
and scarificator on the nape of the neck to remove twelve ounces of blood'.
[3] 'A blistering plaster to be placed behind the ear'.

---

19 July 1841. There is not yet any great improvement.
Repetatur vesicatorum.[1]

1 August 1841. Has had an acute attack of ophthalmia and complains greatly of pain over the eyebrow with photophobia and profuse lachrymation. The sclerotic coat is minutely injected and several red vessels are seen traversing the cornea towards the ulcerated part.
V.S. ad 12 ounces.[2]

An ointment of equal parts of belladonna, opium and blue ointment [a mercury preparation] to be rubbed over the eyebrow. Discontinue the nitrate of silver.

3 August 1841. Less vascularity of the eye and pain abated.
A blister behind the ear.

5 August 1841. The acute attack entirely subdued. The ulcer of the cornea is considerably smaller and she was dismissed with advice.

MALCOLM DAVIDSON, aged 21
St Vigean's parish, Arbroath. A coal miner.
15 June 1841. Admitted to the surgical wards of Professor Syme. He is admitted on account of a conical state of the cornea of both eyes, which has gradually increased since it was first noticed three years ago.

On looking at the eyes, the pupils are seen to be of large size and they do not contract sufficiently on the admission of light. They have a peculiarly clear appearance. The corneas are projecting and have a sparkling appearance and are easily irritated on touching them with a probe. The vision is, as he expresses it, 'dim and misty.' He can read large print with difficulty and can distinguish the number of fingers held before him, or the bars of the window at some distance, but other objects are seen double.

29 June 1841. Dismissed with advice.   R. M.

---

[1] 'Repeat the blistering'.

[2] 'V.S. ad 12 oz.' means 'venesect to twelve ounces'.

PETER MOWAT, age unknown
Shetland. A seaman
1 August 1844. Admitted to surgical wards of Professor Syme. Twenty-eight years since, he received a blow above the right eyebrow in consequence of which the power of vision became gradually diminished in that eye until he could only distinguish light from darkness with it. He had perfect power of vision in the left eye till one year ago when, after exposure to cold, he was attended with violent pain in the forehead extending down to the nose and into the eyeball itself which was much inflamed. It seemed at first as if a fog were spread before his eye and this feeling increased with such rapidity that after three days he was perfectly blind. In this condition he has remained ever since having only the power of distinguishing light from darkness in his left eye.

On examination the right eye is found to be much diminished in size having the appearance, as compared with the left, of being sunk in the head. There is almost no remnant of the iris and the lens is seen white and opaque.

The cornea of the left eye is quite clear but the iris appears to be pushed forward diminishing the extent of the anterior chamber and coming nearer than usual to the cornea. Effusion of lymph has taken place into the iris and the pupil which is much contracted and is occupied by a false membrane.

23 August 1844. Dismissed in *stato quo.*[1]

CHARLES MORRISON, aged 30
Linlithgow, initially from Skye. A quarryman.
10 June 1841. Admitted to surgical wards of Professor Syme on account of inflammation of the eye of five weeks standing, which he refers to no cause rather than that he was working in a quarry and some dust may have entered the eye. He was treated by a surgeon with purgatives. He was bled from the arm and an ointment applied to the eye.

---

[1] This man probably had a traumatic cataract twenty-eight years ago and acute glaucoma one year ago.

On examination the sclerotic and the conjunctiva covering it are congested. The inner margin of the iris is slightly discoloured and there is a little irregularity of the pupil. There is great photophobia and severe frontal headache. The cornea is unaffected.

Applic: hirudines 5 circa orbit.[1] *Habeat haustra cathart.*[2]

16 June 1841. Still complains of frontal headache. The inflammation of the eye unaffected.

Venesect: ad 10 oz.[3]

18 June 1841. Greatly improved. Has very slight headache. Vascularity of the eye much improved.

22 June 1841. Dismissed cured.

[1] Five leeches to be applied around orbit.

[2] To have a catharctic draught.

[3] To have ten ounces of blood removed by venesection.

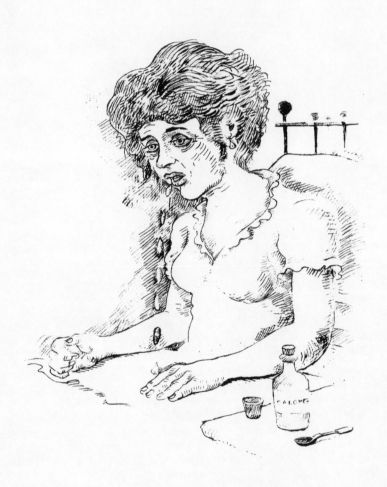

❦ 27 ❦

The Pox

EARL OF SANDWICH 'Pon my soul, Wilkes, I don't know whether you'll
die upon the gallows or of the pox!

WILKES That depends, my Lord, on whether I first embrace
your Lordship's principles or your Lordship's
mistresses!

SIR CHARLES PETRIE in 'The Four Georges'

The cases recorded below are all of syphilis, a common disease of the time, especially with the port of Leith nearby. One case of a post-gonococcal urethral stricture is included elsewhere as an unusual case.

MARY GREEN, aged 32
Leith. A sailor's widow.
20 November 1849. Admitted to ward. Married eight years and has one living child but miscarried the last three pregnancies at three months, two and a half months and six weeks respectively. The first she ascribes to a sudden fright, the second to an accident and the third to her husband's death. None could she ascribe to constitutional causes.

She has suffered from an indolent ulcer of the right leg for the past seven years. About six years ago she was carrying a heavy load of coal up a stair and struck herself on the right hip. Some pustules appeared and healed but others appeared and gave rise to present appearances. She has been in the habit of wading much in the sea. Although she did so in the hope of curing the eruption on the hip, she found it rendered it worse.

On examination numerous ulcerated points grouped together in irregular patches on right hip, extending over six inches by four inches. Individually the ulcers are from a pea to a sixpence. Rounded, with abrupt slightly irregular margins. Flat reddish

---

base with some granulation. The skin round the ulcers is of a copper colour. Between the ulcers are maculae, from a pinhead to a fourpence piece. On the inner right leg at ankle are two ulcerated indolent spots, one to one and a half inches in extent, edges thick and elevated, surrounding skin discoloured. Nil else on examination.

℞ *Calomelanos 1 grain. Sacchar: Alb:* 1 drachm. *Divide in pulv: 12 quorum sumat 1 tid.*[1]

Sores to be dressed with Red lotion and the ulcers on foot strapped and bandaged.[2]

28 November 1849. Ulcer of leg slightly inflamed yesterday with the strapping. Red lotion has been applied and the bandage still continued. The ulcerated parts at the hip are considerably improved, at some point showing symptoms of cicatrisation. Several of them are, however, still open and apparently somewhat inflamed. Patient feels much better but the mouth is slightly sore.

Sumat Pulv: duos tantum in dies[3]

3 December 1849. Mouth quite better.

Sumat pulv: ut antea ter in die[4]

6 December 1849. Mouth continues unaffected. Ulcers of ankle nearly quite recovered – the most superior has entirely cicatrised. Ulcers of hip are improved, in some parts being covered with an

---

[1] 'Calomelanos' is an Edinburgh and Dublin name for the subchloride of mercury, a specific treatment for syphilis. The intention in treatment was to induce the toxic signs and symptoms of mercury poisoning, especially salivation and a sore mouth, and then reduce the dose. There were other uses for mercurials but the phrase 'to be salivated' usually meant 'to be treated for syphilis.' The phrase recurs frequently in the 1840s journals. In this case the mercury was mixed with white (cane) sugar and divided into twelve powders of which one was to be taken three times a day. Salivation could also be induced by the cutaneous application of mercury. Beasley advises this method in children: 'To salivate children, spread diluted mercurial ointment on a flannel roller and place it round one of the child's legs. It cures syphilis without any inconvenience, whereas very few children recover to whom mercury is given internally'.

[2] 'Red lotion' may have been a preparation containing mercuric iodide.

[3] 'To have the powder only twice a day.'

[4] 'To have the powder in the manner as before- three times a day.'

elevated scab, but many have still an angry appearance about the base and edges showing no symptoms of cicatrisation.

Continuentum medicamenti.

25 December 1849. The whole of the ulcers are quite healed and firm cicatrices are perceived over them. She has been completely salivated and has gradually left off taking the powders. It has been ascertained that she was salivated twelve months ago for ulcers on the leg. Dismissed cured.   A. Struthers.

Diagnosis in journal – secondary syphilis.

HENRY CARGILL, aged 20

No fixed abode. Originally from Norfolk. A seaman.

5 August 1844. Admitted to surgical wards of Professor Syme. Two years ago he was admitted to the Newcastle Infirmary in consequence of the swelling of the glands of the right groin which he supposed to result from a venereal disease though he had never observed any sore.

He got a pill three times a day for three weeks. His mouth became sore and his teeth loose but he was not salivated.[1]

The glandular swelling gradually decreased and in five weeks he was dismissed from the Infirmary. Immediately after, he went on a voyage to Hamburgh [*sic*]. Shortly after sailing he was attacked with severe pain in the shoulder and hip joints accompanied by swelling of the left leg and a dull pain in the head. On his return to Newcastle he was so weak that he could hardly move any of his limbs and in this state he was again admitted into the Infirmary. When there, abscesses formed on the forehead and head and glandular swelling took place about the neck and head. He got the decoction of sarsaparilla for seventeen weeks.[2]

---

[1] Salivation-see notes on Mary Green above.

[2] Sarsaparilla was derived from the roots of members of the West Indian plant family smilaceae. The Jamaica sarsaparilla was generally preferred. As was often the case it had many uses but, according to Beasley, 'its advantage is most appreciated in cachectic and depraved conditions of the system, particularly when these depend upon an old venereal disorder' The decoction was produced by 'boiling two and a half ounces of Jamaica Sarsaparilla, cut transversely, in one and a half pints of water for ten minutes and then straining' (BP of 1867).

The abscesses were incised but, as these showed no disposition to heal, he was dismissed as incurable. After this, abscesses formed on the shoulder and breast and he went into the Norwich Infirmary where he remained seven weeks without receiving any other treatment than incision of the abscesses. In May last he went into Bartholomew's Hospital but there he remained only three days after being told that he was not a proper subject for treatment. He afterwards went to his native parish where he was admitted into the workhouse but here also the medical attendant would not interfere with him. Since that time the abscesses in various parts of his body and head have continued open. From those on the head and sternum pieces of bone have on different occasions been discharged.

On examination at present there are found two fistulous openings on the forehead and several on the hairy scalp connected with diseased bone. Over the middle of the sternum is an irregular, crescent shaped patch of ulceration also connected with the bone. The glands of the neck, axilla and groin are swollen and indurated and over each parotid is situated a chronic collection of purulent matter. On his shoulder and neck are several cicatrices of old sores.

To have hydriodate of potass: 2 grains. *Aquae* 1 oz. *Sumat* three times a day.[1] To have a hot bath twice a week.

4 September 1844. Dismissed much improved.

Index of ward journal gives diagnosis as – secondary syphilis.

ALEXANDER BURT, aged 24
Leith. A seaman.
1 August 1844. Admitted to surgical wards of Professor Syme. About a year ago he had a chancre on account of which he took three or four pills each day for two months. At the end of that time he discontinued the medicine, the sore having healed. His mouth was very little affected. After this he continued in his usual health until two months ago when his throat became sore. He paid little

---

[1] Beasley states that the iodide of potassium is 'near specific . . . for secondary syphilis.' Here given three times a day in water.

attention to it at first and it got gradually worse, his voice latterly being so much affected that he cannot speak except in a whisper. He can with difficulty swallow any food being hardly able to open his mouth.

On examination the whole of the fauces is found in a state of ulceration.

To have 1 grain tid of the hydriodide of potassa. The throat to be treated with the nit: argent:[1]

24 August 1844. Dismissed cured.   M.C.

PATRICK TOCHER, aged 33
High School Wynd; Irish. A labourer.
21 June 1841. Admitted to surgical wards of Professor Syme with ulcers on the lower part of each leg and on the posterior aspect of the right thigh. The parts around these sores are swollen and inflamed and they have a hard and a painful base. The edges are raised and thickened and the surface of the sores deep and covered by a slough. These, and similar ones on other parts of the legs, have existed for about twenty months and are probably the result of a venereal affection which he had six years ago and for which he was freely salivated by corrosive sublimate. He says that he took altogether a pennyworth of the salt.[2]

Parts of the arms and legs are covered by a coppery eruption.
℞ *Black wash and a bandage.*[3]
℞ *Hydriod: potass: 1 scruple.*[4] *Aqua* 10 oz. Sol. *Sumat* 1 oz. *bis die.*
19 July 1841. Dismissed cured.   A McK

---

[1] Nit: Argent: is Silver Nitrate

[2] Corrosive sublimate (bichloride of mercury) is a highly toxic compound, a few grains of which are sufficient to cause death.

[3] 'Black wash' was a lotion in which hydrarg: chlor: or calomel (known also in Edinburgh and Dublin as calomelas) was mixed with *aquae calcis* (*liquor calcis* or lime water). It was to be applied to 'indolent and venereal sores' according to a Dr Hooper, quoted by Beasley. In 'yellow wash', bichloride of mercury (corrosive sublimate) replaced the calomel. It was 'to be used externally for syphilitic sores'.

[4] Hydriodide (sometimes referred to as 'hydriodate') of potassium is here given in a dose of one scruple (20 grains) in much water (cf. Cargill and Burt above).

HAMISH CORDINER, aged 24
High Street. A Hackney coachman.
18 June 1845. Admitted to the Infirmary suffering under severe pain in the limbs and a cough of eight weeks duration which arose in consequence of the wet and cold to which he was exposed at work. He is accustomed to the use of a considerable quantity of spirits daily.

He states he had syphilis some years ago but so far as can be ascertained there were no secondary symptoms at that time although he underwent no treatment and went about his work as usual. The sore and the buboes healed up perfectly and he considered himself quite free of the disease. At the same time as the accession of the present complaint, an eruption came out on the whole body for which he was treated by a medical man in town but without success.

Severe pain throughout limbs, the left leg least severely affected. He has much weakness and has been disabled from walking for five weeks. There is no swelling visible about the joints or bones nor are the pains increased by possible collision of the articular surfaces. No pain on compressing the muscular substance of the limbs.

The skin is covered with dark red or copper coloured spots, particularly on the trunk. Those on the arms fainter but equally numerous. There is scarcely any appearance of scales. Auscultation and percussion normal.
℞ *Sumat ter in die tinct: aconite rad: 5 minims ex aqua.*[1]
20 June 1845. No physiological effects.
℞ *Augmentum dos tinct: aconite rad: ad 10 minims ter in die.*[1]

---

[1] 'To have, three times a day, five minims of the tincture of aconite root in water.' Used to relieve pain. Beasley warns of the very poisonous nature of the several preparations of aconite: 'a slight increase in the frequency or strength of the dose may be accompanied by fatal effects. The strength of the pulse must therefore be ascertained before the dose is repeated.' Acotinia, the active principle was too powerful for internal use but was used in ointments e.g. for 'neuralgia.' Beasley warns the prescriber 'to acquaint his patient with its extremely high price, 3s 6p per grain,' and goes on 'we have known this neglected where a quantity of ointment, amounting to several pounds' value, has been ordered'.

21 June 1845. No physiological effects.
℞ *Aug: aconit: ad 15 minims ter in die.*[2]
22 June 1845. Eruption fading. The pains are much better, particularly in left leg.
24 June 1845. Continues improving. Is nearly free of pain. Still slight lameness in right leg.
25 June 1845. Dismissed this day cured.[3]   W. T. G.

[1, 2] As the aconite had no produced no 'physiological' (i.e. toxic) effects the dose was raised to ten and then fifteen minims.

[3] This might just have been a case of tabes dorsalis with 'lightning pains' and difficulty in walking.

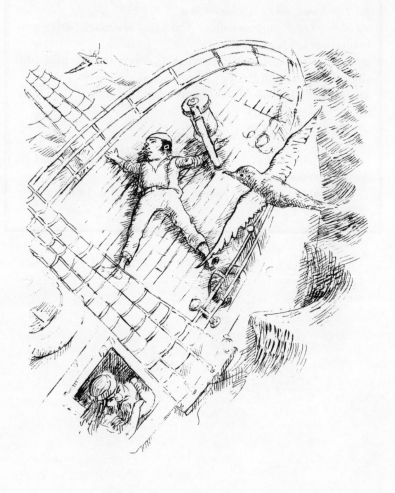

✤ 28 ✤

The Terrible Case of David Brown

Had suffered many things of many physicians ... and
was nothing bettered but rather grew worse.

St Mark

Warning – this Chapter makes uncomfortable reading!
It is difficult to imagine any case in which the treatment given was so
different from that which would have been given today. Late in his
career it is said that Dr Christison, who had looked after Brown for a
time, was beginning to have doubts about the value of removing
blood as a form of treatment. Perhaps Brown's suffering helped him
to this change of view.

David Brown, a professional seaman aged thirty-five years, was
admitted to Edinburgh Royal Infirmary in December 1849. His
birthplace is uncertain but he was probably from Prince Edward
Island in Canada. He also had a connection with Plymouth, England.
He was to remain in the hospital for two and a half years, the first
physicians to look after him being Hughes Bennett and Christison.

---

19 December 1849. Admitted ward 1, Edinburgh Royal Infirmary.
One year ago, at sea, he was struck a severe blow on the back from
the tiller of the vessel. Knocked down and insensible for a short time.
Shortly afterwards he was admitted to Liverpool Infirmary. Leeches
were applied but he was then told that nothing more could be done.
He determined to come to Edinburgh. Mr Bicker-staff of Liverpool
Infirmary later confirmed the above history and said that they had
considered applying galvanism by means of needles passed through
the tumour. This intention was, however, abandoned.[1]

[1] 'Galvanism' was direct elecrical current derived from a chemical battery.
Named after Luigi Galvani 1737–98.

His complaint is of pain in the abdomen and back, and latterly tingling and numbness down the thighs and legs, and prickly pain in the feet especially the left.

On examination he appears strong and active. He is of the bilious temperament. There is an easily visible pulsating tumour in the left hypochondrium, oval, and three inches transversely. The upper end is under the ribs and there is a bellows sound over it. *Diagnosis* – aortic aneurysm.

21 December 1849. Told staff he needs a large dose of morphia to sleep.

℞ *Tinct: Opii* 1½ drachms. *Aqua Font:* 1 oz. *Sumat hora somni*[2]

22 December 1849. No sleep last night. Bled 8 oz.

24 December 1849. Bled 24 oz. No syncope or nausea induced.

25 December 1849. Now has chloroform draught and sleeps better. At his request he now has mutton in place of beef steak, and rice pudding in place of some bread.[3]

26 December 1849. Lies face down to ease the pain.

27 December 1849. Leeches applied.

3 January 1850. Bled 12 oz. No syncope.

22 January 1850. Bled 26 oz. No syncope induced.

25 January 1850. Bled 26 oz. (having been ordered bled again till some faintness or nausea induced.) This time felt faint and skin is pale.

29 January 1850. Bled 10 oz. No syncope. Blister to abdomen.

2 February 1850. Not sleeping.

℞ *Tinct: Cannabis* 15 drops. *Sol. Morph.* ½ oz.[4]

2 February 1850. Not sleeping but pain easier, therefore tonight:

℞ *Tinct: Cannabis. Sol: Morph.* each ½ oz.

5 February 1850. No sleep, pain +.

℞ *Enema with Liq: Opii 40 minims sedat.*

6 February 1850. No sleep, but best relief of pain so far.

8 February 1850. Bled 20 oz. Fainted, quick recovery.

[2] 'To have at hour of sleep', i.e. at bedtime.

[3] The board of management had requested staff to prescribe only the hospital's fixed diets but this patient, possibly by virtue of his 'old salt's' skill, managed to achieve variations.

[4] '*Gtt*' means '*guttae*' or 'drops'. One drop is one minim.

2 March 1850. Bled 14 oz. No syncope.

Piles– apply *Ung: Gallae et Opii.*[5]

10 March 1850. Bled 23 oz. No syncope.

19 March 1850. Bled 8 oz.

6 April 1850. Bled 13 oz.

15 April 1850. Took a walk in the open air but felt rather the worse for it.

21 April 1850. Bled 34 oz. at his own urgent request. Admitted feeling nothing until all that quantity had flowed when he fell over in a state of syncope and was with some difficulty revived. His appearance is now very anaemic, his tongue pale and marked by the teeth. Pulse slow and feeble. Feels very weak.

30 April 1850. Still very weak. Blood removed on 21 April contained in 10,000 parts: dry globules – 600; solids of serum – 823; dry fibre – 31; water – 8564.[6]

5 May 1850. Pulsation much less but bruit still heard. Complains of shooting pains down the back between the shoulders and down the arms. Cannot sleep without a morphia draught. Does not like eggs and diet altered as follows: breakfast – 1 biscuit (1½ oz.), tea – 10 oz.; dinner – 2 biscuits (2½ oz.), calf foot jelly (4 oz.); tea – 1 biscuit (1½ oz.), tea 10 oz.

22 May 1850. Still complains of back pain relieved by the enema with *Sol: Mur: Morph:* which he takes every night.

30 May 1850. Continues the opiate injection ['injection' meant 'enema' at this time.]

1 June 1850. Has had much pain in the tumour for past three days and shooting upwards and downwards. The opiate injection seems to give no relief now.

Applic: hirud: VIII parte dolente and to have 20 drops of Jeremy's solution daily.[7]

---

[5] Lead and opium ointment.

[6] Brown had now been bled 11 pints (i.e. 8.4 litres) in the four months from 22 December to 21 April. In addition leeches had been applied at least six times in the same period. The present practice of the Scottish Blood Transfusion Service is to bleed donors to less than half of one litre (480 ml.) at a time and never oftener than once in three months. There was no modern indication for venesection in Brown's case at any time.

[7] Jeremy's solution [not traced].

17 June 1850. Still very weak. Less pain. Moves about the ward with crutches. Now has meat in place of calf foot jelly.

28 June 1850. Complains at 11 am of pain and pulsation in the tumour which was much larger. But much better in 2–3 hours and the tumour had returned to its former condition, i.e. barely prominent above the surface.

1 July 1850. Much better again.

8 July 1850. Is able to walk a little in the open air but with a good deal of pain.

17 July 1850. Applic: hirudines XII parte dolente.[8]

30 July 1850. Is considerably stronger now and can walk better.

7 August 1850. Several small haemorrhoids give him great uneasiness and prevent him using the injection pipe [the enema apparatus].

Ordered Ung: Gallae et opii.

9 August 1850. Easier, and could use injection last night

12 August 1850. Still c/o uneasiness of piles and pain of tumour. *Inject: opii b.d.* and apply iced water.[9]

Applic: hirudines duodecim parte dolente.[10]

17 August 1850. Was so weak and faint after the leeches that he was ordered two ounces of wine and the opiate injection at night.

19 August 1850. No relief from cold water.

To have *Sol. opiat: sedat:* (Batley) minims 4 when the pain increases.[11]

30 August 1850. Out yesterday for one hour on pass. Since then complains of pain in the abdomen and back and latterly tingling and numbness down the thighs and legs and prickly pain in the feet especially the left.

14 September 1850. Goes out once a week on pass and is able to take a good deal of exercise without causing pain or increased pulsation. Does not require the opiate enema so often.

---

[8] 'Apply eight leeches to the painful part'.

[9] 'Inject.' here should be '*injict.*' meaning '*injiciatur enema*' or, as Beasley says, 'Let a clyster be given.'

[10] 'Apply twelve leeches to the painful part.'

[11] Also known as 'liquor opii sedativus' (Batley), the dose being 5–20 minims.

16 September 1850. More pain.

Applic: hirud: XII parte dolente.

19 September 1850. Has been unable to leave his bed on account of great weakness since the last bleeding.

24 September 1850. Has greatly recovered his strength; is able to be up but does not leave the ward.

20 October 1850. Pain still severe in tumour.

Applic: hirud: VIII parte dolente

23 October 1850. No abatement of the pain. Takes 60 drops of the Batley's solution and 40 of Jeremy's with very little effect on pain while it causes griping pain and numbness of legs but no tendency to sleep.

℞ *Tartaris Antimonii* 3 grains. *Sumat* 2 drachms [illegible] *singulis dosibus opiati.*[12]

24 October 1850. The antimony seemed only to have the effect of making him more restless and was abandoned.

Ordered 3 drops of Cajeput oil at night.[13]

25 October 1850, The tumour was observed to be movable today. When he lies on his left side the prominence is concealed by the cartilages of his left ribs but it moves three to four inches to the right side when he lies on his back, above and a little to the right of his umbilicus. This he states has been the case for the past week. Previous to that it had been stationary.

28 October 1850. Complains the Cajeput oil burns him but took last night ten drops along with the opiate enema and felt much relieved.

20 November 1850. He has suffered since the period of the last report much less than previously though during the last week he has complained of a sharp pain under the left clavicle for which he was ordered six leeches.

22 November 1850. The pain not being eased he was ordered to be cupped which was repeated today.[14]

---

[12] Antimony had many uses. The indication for it here is unclear.

[13] Cajeput Oil was distilled from the leaves of the plant Melaleuca Minor which was imported from Singapore and Batavia (Jakarta). Used for colic, amongst other things.

[14] Further iatrogenic blood loss.

27 December 1850. Has continued much the same but lately has complained of sharp pain in the tumour. Bled to eight ounces with considerable relief.

17 February 1851. Has continued in same condition and having had considerable pain was again bled to 6 oz.

20 February 1851. For the last four months he has been on the following diet: Breakfast – 1 roll, Dinne r– wing of a fowl and two potatoes, Supper – 1 roll. Wine: four ounces daily. On auscultation the blowing murmur now inaudible and the tumour feels more solid and the size of a pigeon's egg or rather larger.

30 March 1851. Complains of pain. Venesect 6 ounces.

31 March 1851. Much relieved by v.s. [*sic*].

2 April 1851. Bled 12 oz.

3 April 1851. The pain not being relieved he has been ordered a blister.

13 April 1851. Complained of severe pain in the tumour. Opiate injection at bedtime as before.

15 April 1851. Pain continues.

℞ *Tinct: Cannabis Indica minims 36. Aqua Fontana 3 oz. Sumat 1 oz. tert: qqh.*[15] *Repetitur enema opiat.*

17 April 1851. Pain much abated.

2 May 1851. Severe pain. Bled to six ounces with relief.

28 May 1851. Pain.

℞ *Injiciatur Enema Amylii cum Sol: Morph: 2 oz.*[16]

30 May 1851. Pain. Leeches 12.

1 June 1851. Very little relief followed the leeching.

Applicatur dorso cucurbitula cruenta ut mittetur sang: oz. 6.[17]

5 June 1851. Pain continues.

Applic: cucurb: cruent: ut mittetur sang: oz. 5.

8 June 1851. Complains of pain as much as ever.

Mittetur sang: oz. 12.[18]

11 June 1851. Pain much relieved since last bleeding.

---

[15] 'Every third hour.'

[16] 'To have an enema of Starch and Morphine.'

[17] 'To be cupped (including the use of the scarificator), on the back, removing six ounces of blood.'

[18] Yet more induced blood loss.

24 June 1851. Pain again being the same he was this day cupped to eight ounces with very little relief.

25 June 1851. Pain. *Leeches 14.*

26 June 1851. Pain has undergone very little abatement since cupping and leeching. He has therefore been ordered to be bled from the arm to twelve ounces.

27 June 1851. Much relieved.

29 October 1851. Since last report the symptoms have continued as formerly. The bleeding has occasionally been resorted to when pain severe. Diet at present is: Breakfast – 1 roll and 1 pint of tea. Dinner– 1 flounder and two potatoes. Supper – 1 roll and 1 pint of tea. 3 ounces of brandy daily.

31 October 1851. Generally pain for an hour or two after rising in the morning. Appetite good.

4 November 1851. Comfortable this morning. Pain always oppressive after rising for a few hours.

23 November 1851. Yesterday much difficulty in voiding the urine, not from any obstruction but from general weakness.

℞ *Decoct: Scoparii* oz. 6.[19] *Aetheris Nitrici* drachms 1½. Two tablespoonfuls three times a day.[20]

29 November 1851. There has been since last report great weakness; there is difficulty in making water from great muscular debility. Occasional bleeding from piles.[21]

12 December 1851. Complains of great pain in site of tumour. *Leeches 12.*

Cough troublesome.

℞ *Tinct: Opii Ammoniat:* oz. ½. *Syrupi Scillae* [illegible]. *Acac:* drachms 1. *Aq. Menthae* oz. ½. One tablespoonful three times a day.[22]

15 December 1851. Relief of pain after leeches .

21 December 1851. Cough easier. Pain as before.

---

[19] Scoparius is broom, the fresh tops of which have a diuretic action (Beasley).

[20] The tablespoonful was by this time beginning to be used as a unit of dose measurement.

[21] More blood loss.

[22] A syrup made from scilla bulbs, a plant 'growing on the coast of the Mediterranean' according to Beasley, and also known as squill.

15 January 1852. Tumour about size of a walnut. Great weakness and feeling of numbness in left side and considerable pain in right leg. Walking much more difficult. Continues the morphia injection. Appetite good.

Blood oz. 8 to be taken from the arm.

16 January 1852. Easier since abstraction of blood but the pain was oppressive this morning so the opiate injection was taken.

19 January 1852. Weakness very great. Bowels costive.

℞ *Pil. Colocynth comp.* scruples 2. *Extr. Hyoscyami scruples 1. Misce et divide in pilulas XII. Sumat unam vel duas pro re nata.*[23]

23 January 1852. As at last report. Appetite bad. A little milk and bread is all his food. Pulse feeble. Continues the opiate injection every morning.

29 January 1852. On Saturday last felt much coldness over the whole body but there was no distinct rigor. Left side and shoulder painful. Complete dullness on whole of left side. Respiration is feeble and intermittent over the whole of the left side and at some points inaudible. Bronchophony is heard posteriorly where it is of aegophonic character. No creps. Cough and spit severe but no blood expectorated. Great weakness and loss of appetite. Pulse small, feeble

℞ *Pulv: Opii* grains 1. *Pulv: Aromat:* grains 3 [24]

30 January 1852. Respiration more audible but no expectoration. Warm fomentations were attended with great relief.

℞ *Vin: Ipecac:* drachms ½. *Sol: Morph:* drachms 2. *Mist:* [illegible] oz. 6. *Sumat* [illegible][25]

2 February 1852. Sputum slightly tinged with blood.

4 February 1852. Cough relieved. Has not slept well for two nights. Complete aegophony. Less sputum and less blood-tinged. Slight friction to left of left nipple.

[23] Colocynth is a purgative, the added hyoscyamus possibly for relief of the spasm of purgation. The instruction reads: 'Mix and divide into twelve pills. To have one or two as required.'

[24] 'Pulv. Aromat.' (Aromatic Powder of Chalk) contained cinnamon, nutmeg, cloves and cardamom, with saffron, refined sugar and chalk.

[25] From the clinical note, ipecacuanha probably being used here for its supposed expectorant effect. Beasley says it has 'a specific effect on the bronchial mucous membrane so as to excite its secretion when it is too dry.'

7 February 1852. Still left chest pain with shooting pain in shoulder. Dullness and friction unchanged.

8 February 1852. Habeat Emplastrum Cantharidis 4 x 5 lateri sinistro.[26]

10 February 1852. Pain considerably alleviated by blister.

16 February 1852. Slight motion observed on left side during respiration. Dullness slightly diminished below left clavicle.

20 February 1852. From being in the habit lately of taking Calomel and Jalapa as a purgative, he has been profoundly salivated and his gums are very tender and partially ulcerated.[27]

℞ *Calcis Chlorinat: drachm I. Aqua oz.6. Fiat gargarisma, saepe utendum.*[28]

1 March 1852. Friction is heard all over the left chest posteriorly and at the apex of the lung anteriorly. Dullness rapidly diminishing and there is considerable respiratory movement on left side. Cough quite gone. His lower limbs have been for a time almost powerless but sensation is unimpaired in them. He has a very troublesome bedsore which has been much relieved by poultices. A large slough seems about to separate from the sacral region. There is no perceptible change in the size of the aneurismal tumour nor in the force of its pulsations. The wash which he was ordered for his mouth has completely cured the soreness of his gums.

8 March 1852. Now no signs of pleurisy. The slough on the sacrum has separated.

8 April 1852. His limbs are quite paralysed from the upper part of the thigh. The powers of sensation and motion are both lost. He cannot lie on his back nor sit up for the tenderness of the sacrum and the sores on that region. He has not suffered so much from the aneurism latterly and the pulsations are not so strong. Bruit still heard. He is much troubled by twitching and starting of the paralysed limbs. The morphia injection is given every morning which relieves the aneurism pain.

---

[26] This blistering plaster, made from cantharis (a dried beetle, 'Spanish fly'). measuring four by five inches, was to be applied to the left side [? of the chest].

[27] These are toxic effects of Mercury (here administered as Calomel).

[28] 'Make a gargle to be used often.'

31 May 1852. Today he was poisoned by taking a quantity of a liniment containing aconite. He died in about five minutes. No change in his condition had occurred for many months. For post mortem appearances see pathologist's book.[29]

Extract from Edinburgh pathological register, Vol.14, No. 437
Clinical Summary. David Brown, aged 35, had been two years in No.1 being treated for an abdominal aneurism. Poisoned himself with aconite. Had latterly complete paraplegia.
Pathological findings A male, pale and sallow, somewhat emaciated. About thirty-five years of age.

Right lung shows miliary tubercle in upper lobe and some miliary lesions in middle and lower lobes. Left lung somewhat compressed posteriorly but otherwise apparently normal. Is attached at the posterior part of the lower lobe to a large sacculated tumour in front of the dorsal vertebrae arising from the descending aorta. It is also attached to the bodies of several vertebrae which can be felt to be extremely eroded and destroyed. The tumour is flaccid but if distended would equal in size a moderate sized coconut. The pancreas is stretched over an abdominal tumour about the size of a small coconut [at this point there is a marginal note by W. T. Gairdner, the Pathologist to the Infirmary: 'Very small coconut. Seems about four inches in length in its largest diameter.'] movable in front of the aorta and tolerably resistant and firm. It seems to be attached to some of the great vessels and to the abdominal aorta itself.

The dorsal and part of the lumbar spine, two or three inches of the ribs, the heart, aorta, part of the trachea and oesophagus, left lung, stomach, duodenum, pancreas and both tumours and the neighbouring parts were removed en masse for further examination and sent to the University (care of Dr Cobbold). Other organs normal i.e. liver, spleen, intestine, kidneys.
Summary of pathological findings Thoracic and abdominal aneurisms. Tubercle, partly obsolete, partly recent and miliary in right lung.

---

[29] This man's life and his clinical notes both ended abruptly!

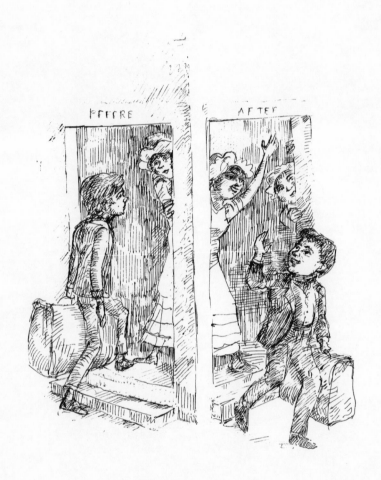

Afterword

Edinburgh's hospital and dispensary services were predictably excellent in mid-Victorian times; I have not discovered anywhere else as universally available a medical service as that given by the Royal Infirmary and its doctors.

Geoffrey Best, *Mid-Victorian Britain*

This is real praise coming as it does from Professor Best, a historian with a special interest in Victorian Britain. Surgically the hospital was known far and wide as efficient. Medically it was as good as any, at a time when there were few effective medicines. Although it was firm in its handling of patients and staff, Edinburgh Royal Infirmary was also a kindly place. There are several examples in this book of its sympathetic approach, the Widow Cossar, for example, being generously dealt with by the board.

One six-year old, admitted at a low point in his short life, was much the better of his stay. His Christian name has not been changed.

HERCULES McFARLANE, AGED 6
Address not recorded.
28 September 1849. Admitted thin and of sickly appearance.
24 October 1849. Improved much under the use of a generous diet. Sleeps with a hyoscyamus draught.
3 December 1849. General condition good, and appears now stout. Discharged cured.

This boy had no long-term clinical problem. His malnutrition was cured by the Infirmary's 'generous diet' and he was allowed to stay long enough in the comfort of the ward for his improvement to become obvious. One can almost hear the nurses' laughter down the years as the now more appropriately built Hercules left the hospital, ready to tackle such labours as might lie ahead of him.

Bibliography

'A Medical Gentleman', *Low Life in Victorian Edinburgh*, Paul Harris, 1980, an edited version of *An Enquiry into Destitution, Prostitution and Crime in Edinburgh*, Edinburgh, 1851

Anderson, John, *History of Edinburgh from the Earliest Period to the Completion of the Half-century, 1851)*, Fullarton, Edinburgh and London, 1856

Bailey, Hamilton, *Notable Names in Medicine and Surgery*, H. K. Lewis, London, 1983

Beasley, Henry, *The Book of Prescriptions*, John Churchill, London, 1854

Belloc, Hilaire, 'Henry King' in *Cautionary Verses*, published by Random House (UK Ltd) per Peters, Fraser and Dunlop, Writers' Agents, London

Best, Geoffrey, *Mid-Victorian Britain: 1851–1875*, Weidenfeld and Nicolson, 1985

British Medical Journal

Christison, Sir Robert, *The Life of Sir Robert Christison, Bart.*, Edited by his sons, Blackwood, Edinburgh and London, 1886

Crew, F. A. E., In *Scientific Survey of South East .Scotland*, British Association for the Advancement of Science, 1951

Edinburgh Pathological Register, in Lothians Health Services Archive, Edinburgh University Library

Exotic Disease Series, No 6, pp. 17–20, British Ministry of Agriculture, 1995

Gibson, George, *The Life of Sir W. T. Gairdner*, Maclehose, Glasgow. 1910

Kauffman, Professor Matthew, 'Cut to the Bone', *Edit, Issue 12*, Edinburgh University, 1997

Bibliography

The Lancet

Lloyd and Coulter, *Medicine in the Navy:* 1200-1900, Vol. 3, 1714–1815, Livingstone, Edinburgh

Minute Books of Board of Management of the Royal Infirmary of Edinburgh 1840–49 in Lothians Health Services Archive, Edinburgh University Library

Scottish Medical Journal (Extracts from the journal under its previous titles of *Edinburgh Medical Journal, Edinburgh Medical and Surgical Journal,* etc.

Scott, R. F., *The Voyage of the* Discovery, John Murray, London, 1905

Shepherd, John, *Simpson and Syme of Edinburgh,* Livingstone Edinburgh, 1969

Simpson, Myrtle, *Simpson the Obstetrician,* Gollancz, London, 1972

Stewart, Professor Grainger. Sketch *of the History of Edinburgh Royal Infirmary and of the Development of Clinical Teaching,* Volume 1 of Edinburgh Hospital Reports

Sidney, S., *The Book of the Horse,* Cassell, Petter and Galpin (first published more than one hundred years ago).

The British Pharmacopoeia, 1867

The History and Statutes of the Royal Infirmary of Edinburgh, The Authorities, 1778

Thomson, A. T., *Elements of Materia Medica and Therapeutics.* Longman, Rees, Orme, Brown, Green and Longman, London, 1835

Ward Journals of Edinburgh Royal Infirmary, 1840–49, in Lothians Health Services Archive, Edinburgh University Library

Yule. W. L., 'In search of a medical artist', *The Lancet,* 5 September 1998.

Sources

Full details of each source will be found in the bibliography. Almost all the chapters contain material from the minute books, ward journals and pathological records of the Royal Infirmary. Additional sources for each chapter are listed below.

CHAPTER 1
Stewart, Professor Grainger.
The History and Statutes of the Royal Infirmary of Edinburgh.

CHAPTER 2
Edinburgh Medical Journal

CHAPTER 4
Bailey, Hamilton
Shepherd, John
Lancet
Edinburgh Medical Journal

CHAPTER 6
Christison, Sir R.
Edinburgh Medical Journal

CHAPTER 7
Edinburgh Medical Journal

CHAPTER 8
Shepherd, John
Simpson, Myrtle

CHAPTER 9
The British Pharmacopoeia
Christison, Sir R.
Edinburgh Medical Journal

CHAPTER 10
Lloyd and Coulter
Scott, R. F

CHAPTER 11
'A Medical Gentleman'
Anderson, John

CHAPTER 12
Crew, F. A. E.
Gibson, George
Edinburgh Medical Journal

CHAPTER 15
Gibson, George
Yule, W. L.

CHAPTER 16
The Lancet
Edinburgh Medical Journal

CHAPTER 17
Sidney, S
Exotic Disease Series
Edinburgh Medical Journal

CHAPTER 18
Anderson, John

CHAPTER 19
Thomson, A. T.
The British Pharmacopoeia.

CHAPTER 21
Kauffman, Professor M.
Shepherd, John

AFTERWORD
Best, Professor Geoffrey